Sober & Fabulous

How the courage to give up
alcohol transforms the way we
look, eat and succeed.

Rebecca Sweeney

DEDICATION

This book is dedicated to anybody who has had a struggle. Any person who has had a struggle or road block in life that is so debilitating they do not know if they can get out of bed in the morning. These are incredible conversations dedicated to anyone feeling so painful with guilt, they do not know if they can ever forgive themselves. This book is for the people who do not know if they can ever talk about their past. This is for my kindred spirits who are embarrassed of their weight, or feel disgusted with their body. This is for all the people who are embarrassed of their choices.

I dedicate these words in this book, from start to finish, to the 30-somethings who have felt pathetic in their drinking habits that have developed over time. I dedicate this to anyone who has struggled either with an excessive weight or struggled with an eating disorder. This book is for my lovely sisters or brothers who have had discomfort in their mind or body that has been so strong they're not sure there's a solution for them.

CONTENTS

ACKNOWLEDGMENTS

I would be nowhere without the support of my husband and my soldier. He is a constant inspiration to me, has supported me so much in my coaching career and is an incredible, humorous and creative father to our girls.

I do have to give props to a man named Lee M. Jenkins who runs a great Facebook business page. He was the first person who told me to write a book.

A friend of mine, Claire Louise Hay is a spiritual teacher and healing guidance coach in Australia. She's sort of, a wellness-business mastermind friend of mine. She wrote a book and she inspires me in my own business.

I have to say a huge shout out to teammate business partner of mine, drummer and high school mate, Eric James Danowski who was the last person I spoke to before I quit drinking alcohol. He was one of the people who really made me see the light when sobriety was too scary and abstract for me to imagine considering. But I did it, in part, because of him and his guidance, spirit and own clean life. He is awesome.

And I have to acknowledge every single last customer and friend of mine on my fitness team, Team Flourish, *they* are who teach me daily and inspired me to write a book and give me the spark to want to continue helping people.

"If Americans do not change their eating and drinking habits within twenty years we will have nutritional obliteration."

Dr. James Beasley
Ford Foundation Project
http://www.danreid.org/health-alerts-sour-dough-health.asp

Chapter 1
YOU WANT ME TO WHAT?

I am not going to rip off the band aid of your life's comfort blankets. I am not going to tell you to stop drinking your alcohol and coffee. But what I am going to tell you are the absolutely extraordinary and fabulous things that happened to me and some other good people when our life's choices and journeys lead us to living sober.

When I sat down to write this book, my goal was to keep it simple. I planned to put into print the best and most common subject matters I have learned for myself in my wellness and weight loss roller coaster of a journey. I was going to put the tips and tricks I heard myself saying over and over and over every day to customers and friends into a workbook for those going through their own weight loss journey. "Put it all in a book! Great idea," I thought. A book would be something solid to give to my awesome customers in my fitness coaching business. Also I knew my partners in this life, in the process of their own, who might be able to utilize a hard copy of my advice to hold onto and refer back to. Currently I have lost nearly all of the 60 pounds I set out to lose. I am doing pretty well and people really do constantly struggle with weight loss. "I sure do have something to share," I thought. "My team of coaches is growing and I am a leader," I thought. "I **do** have the skills to do this book!" But when my writing process began, the process itself very quickly, dramatically and quite Divinely ripped the rug from under my confident feet. I began creating, and my book turned from weight loss or fitness to a much, much scarier and foreign subject. I often say nowadays, that I no longer sat to write a book, the book just started being written through me.

In sitting to "write a book," I knew I was no journalist or writer. I felt far, far away from my creative writing classes in college, but still I desperately wanted a workbook for my customers to be made. I was lead to seek counsel on how to write a book of this nature and I took a class. In this non-fiction publishing workshop, I was recommended to interview certain people to help my book along and to have them contribute to the process, to help the development and thoughts that were in my head already, to have people to quote in the book, etc. So I thought about my "weight loss and wellness" book long and hard. I thought about the people who I looked up to the most in health and wellness matters, the people who I knew throughout my experiences who were the picture of goals met, with a healthy body, and a balanced life. For some reason, the people who I found who I wanted to interview turned out to be all people who happened to *not* drink alcohol, ever. They just did not ever drink! I noticed after I compiled my "hope to interview" list, I looked up to them for that aspect of their lives. *That* was the picture of cleanliness and health in my mind, apparently. I did not understand this totally until my list had formed. This list made me look at my own life, my goals and my own alcohol intake. For some reason, alcohol became something dirty to me over the past few years. The healthier and healthier I became in my most recent fitness and weight loss mission, the more and more I just really wanted to give up alcohol all together. But... not so easy.

I never considered myself to wear the textured title of "alcoholic." But why was drinking so hard for me to give up forever then? I struggled with this friction in my head. I struggled with the "forever" word and with the thought of NEVER drinking again. Questions started drowning my brain: "Why did I have to commit to forever? Whenever I try to quit, why do I cave in, when offered a drink? When others are around me drinking heavily, why do I start to guzzle?" These tests would always inevitably happen when I was trying to break from alcohol. And with drink in hand, I would quietly think to myself, "What happened to taking a temporary alcohol break?" Then entered into my brain that creepy word again: forever.

More so than those irritating ideas, I struggled with wine as an artistic ritual and a thing of beauty to me. I also struggled with an "off switch," so to speak. Once I started drinking, with just one glass of a fine red pinot, I could never just stop and enjoy it for what it was. More often than not, I had no off switch. And usually one glass of wine would lead to a bottle. And if I broke out the cocktails on a special occasion, I could probably put away a good 4-8 stiff ones, no problem. Here's the thing, I was not stumbling or cursing or puking after that either. I just felt sort of numb in my last few years of consuming. I maybe got a little louder, sometimes said or did something really inappropriate and overly silly. But in my adult life, I never really got smashed. In my thirties drinking was an ongoing and endless life style or, dare I say, habit. The nights I allowed myself to drink were actually very uneventful. No more fun. No more wild, loud parties, bar hopping, socializing and music and dancing and twirling about. No. It was sad, kids in bed, on the couch, drinking. Or if I did make it out to the occasional special girls night, it was sitting, fat butt on a bar stool and racking up hundreds of dollars. Shots, beers, wine and drinks, only to end the Jack Handy-esque conversations of searching our souls and figuring out our deep meanings of bad choices made. Talking about what our lives delivered us and where we had gone wrong was what we called fun in the 30's. We would find our way home one way or another, go to bed too late, only to get up too early to feed the too noisy kids and feel like dirt for most of the next day. Wild. Crazy. Wow. Awesome. Fun. Glamorous, right?

It simply was not working for me anymore. I questioned drinking in my thirties ever since the age of about 29. I looked at people who did not drink alcohol and their lives seemed spectacular, fruitful. I had a gut instinct to ask a good friend from college, named Jamila, why and how she did it. After reconnecting with her many years post-college, on social media, I straight up emailed her, "How and why did you stop drinking?" She told me her story and I vaguely remember it seemed to revolve around her yoga instructing. Funny thing, I was a yoga instructor for going on 10 years at that time and I had never had the inclination to quit; not for my stomach problems, not for balancing my chi, prana or any other reason! She inspired me and I had no idea why. It wasn't about the yoga, it was about the love of self she had, that I was lacking, clearly.

More recently, I had heard from an old friend, traveling through town, that a really interesting guy who we knew in grade school, named Travis, had quit drinking. And the meaningless side comment on a "catching up" conversation, stuck in my brain about him, and I wondered why he had made that choice? At the origin of this nagging thought, I never realized, a few months later, I would be interviewing him and really feeling like God was working through me, no really, *SHOUTING* through me.

But for as long as I can remember, an old colleague and business partner of mine named David, who I knew from my past affiliation with a nutrition company, did not drink alcohol. I was not sure why, but he for sure was a picture of what I assumed perfection was in health. He was a vital, kind, happy, surfer, wealthy home-based business owner, smoothie every day and traveling every year-kinda' guy and I also knew that he was alcohol free. He was the guru in my head, what perfect health and balanced life looked like.

My list got to about four to six people long. So I started out to call only *these* people for interviews for some reason. I felt somewhat of a lingering struggle with my idea of quitting alcohol. And if I was going to walk the walk and talk the talk of a wellness coach writing a book, I thought maybe I could try and *not* drink alcohol like them. It was a fine idea to me because I felt I had conquered yoga, fitness, nutrition and over all life style balance in every single way, except two places: marriage, and alcohol. I set out to fix these things. -And fix them full force, all in, 100%. The result of these interviews **drastically** changed the way I was writing my book. This book was going to be suggesting people think, embrace and just merely toss around the idea of living a life alcohol free, -alcohol abusers or not! I am simply suggesting, very profoundly, that we all take a good, hard look at the way we celebrate, we dine, we holiday, we exercise and we live. I quit drinking for myself about three to four weeks before these interviews started. I was still on the fence if this was going to be a finite decision for me.

In my non-fiction book writing workshop, I was told to pick a partner, who was a stranger to me, to interview me regarding the subject matter of my book. This Q and A would then become a developing transcript and guideline for my eventual book. A book expert who I spoke with after the workshop, suggested I just keep the book in that Q and A format, because he felt not nearly enough books were written in this way. It all fell in line with the magic interviews I held, so I liked the idea, everything started forming really naturally, the book just unfolded. So, please know that the remainder of this book is my organic, free flowing conversation on how my life shockingly, dramatically, Divinely and very surprisingly changed after interviewing my friends who all live their lives totally alcohol free. To contribute more to this book's direction, I interviewed a few people to expand on a testimonial they had given me in the past for my web site on my teaching and coaching and their experiences with it. These randomly picked customers and friends told me, as we expanded their on testimonials in interviews, that each of them was also alcohol free. I had had no earthly idea that these kind customers were living their lives alcohol free as well. My mind was officially blown. All of a sudden, *they* became my teachers. Their interviews expanded to be much more than testimonials! Those incredible conversations fall at the end of the book and brought a beautiful and amazing, full circle, blessing of an experience to me, as the writer. But they also made me see, this book was not forming coincidentally and was not about me or my coaching at all. It was all meant to spread this one, pure message to the world.

Once completed, my initial interviews immediately changed my plans. They became the new sole purpose, total direction, and beginning of the book. The first three incredible interviews I held shook me in their words, stories, experiences and most importantly, in their drastic similarities. They changed me. These first people did not know one another and were from three very different places and experiences when their stories and sober lives began. My journey is told after and in gratitude to those who have bravely shared their intimate stories with me and all of us. Please don't think this book is about depriving yourself of anything at all, but rather, just let yourself open up to the beauty that has been shown to me and exists for you. I merely wish to share the spectacular Grace with you. I expect you will do with it what you see fit.

CHAPTER 2
THE DIVINE INTERVIEWS
(The First Three)

We will start off in this journey, by sharing with you the first 3 interviews I held, in their specific order, in the preparation of building material for this book:

Interview #1
David McLaughlin, founder of www.club100k.com, Boulder, CO

Q. Rebecca: When did you quit drinking alcohol?

A. David: August 27th, 1992 was when I quit everything. I was 22 years old.

Q. Rebecca: Why did you decide to quit drinking and/or using substances?

A. David: I quit because of my abuse of using all drugs and alcohol. I was drinking/abusing since I was 15 years old. I lead the rock star life style.

Q. Rebecca: What brought you to the place of saying, "I quit this all?"

A. David: I had been using meth, coke, alcohol, all of it and this time around was for about 2 weeks straight. I was touring with the Grateful Dead and friends. I remember I was taking a box out to load up a car and I felt like I was starting to lose it mentally, after being on this 2 week binge. All at once I felt myself start to lose it. But then, I had a moment of sobriety hit me. I heard a voice. I heard God speak to me. It was like an out of body experience. I heard the voice say, "you cannot get any higher, that's it. You cannot get any higher. This is it. Enough." And that's it. I quit then, 100%.

Q. Rebecca: Wow. I did not know that was why you gave up alcohol, etc. I thought it was always just a personal choice you made in wellness. Ever since I've known you over 10 years now, I just always thought that you just didn't drink. So immediately after you quit it all, how did you feel?

A. David: After quitting, you know a sense of pride came with sobriety. Then it was challenging. I did NA (Narcotics Anonymous) and I just felt it was so limiting.

Q. Rebecca: How did you feel it was limiting?

A. David: Well you know, they tell you not to hang out with the people you always knew, or do the things you always did. And I was not ok with that. So, I continued on touring with the Grateful Dead and I was fine sober. I got to travel 40 states throughout my 20's. You know, I would never change that experience.

Q. Rebecca: So you had no trouble like, not drinking at a bar with your same old friends?

A. David: Right after I quit, it was hard for me at a bar. I did feel uncomfortable at a bar, there were times where I was sober at a bar and just had to leave because I was like, shaking.

Q. Rebecca: How do you feel today?

A. David: I am 42 now. I feel great now! Life is great.

Q. Rebecca: When offered a drink now, how do you handle that? Or what do you say?

A. David: When I am offered a drink, I just say, "I don't drink anymore." Or I say, "no thank you, I don't drink."

Q. Rebecca: Yea, I think it is a shame that we all celebrate every holiday and wedding with alcohol or a "bar" involved. If you sit at a fine restaurant, you are immediately given a wine list. I want people to start to question or think about this. How do you feel in social or celebratory situations being alcohol free?

A. David: Drinking, it's socially acceptable and highly addictive. Yeah. I still have friends that party, friends that are sober and friends that drink, etc. You know, it is fine, it is not a big deal. As far as the wine lists in restaurants, I think it is like any other business, it is economical, a money maker. But, I think your book topic about living alcohol free, it is a good thing to look at, for sure.

Interview #2
Travis
Q. Rebecca: When did you quit drinking alcohol?

A. Travis: The decision to quit was in December of '07 to January of '08.

Q. Rebecca: Why did you decide to quit drinking alcohol?

A. Travis: I went to Dennison and lived the typical college lifestyle. There was drinking, daily weed, you know the whole thing. Then, I moved to Charleston which has a big drinking, beach culture, but then I started to notice that I drank more than my friends. Later down the road I got work in D.C. and got engaged. I was working, I would go home for lunch and drink a 6 pack. Then I would go back to work. I realized I was a totally functioning alcoholic. I called off the marriage. I moved back home. Once home, I realized that when I drank, 90% of the time, I was drinking against my will. And I realized then it was an addiction.

But then one night I had a moment of clarity. I was driving home from work on a Friday. I had been drinking all day. I damn near blacked out. And then all of a sudden I had like, 2 seconds of sobriety, I moment of sobriety and I heard a voice. It was from outside of me, like God or something, it said, "Enough." Over and over I kept hearing, "this is enough, no more. You cannot do this anymore." I knew I could not get another D.U.I. and I just realized this had to stop. And I decided to go to treatment.

Q. Rebecca: How did you feel immediately after you made the decision to be sober?

A. Travis: In treatment, you know you feel amazing. But there is a full range of emotions: "I love it, never felt better, self-pity, bad days." But after the first year, it really feels like, this is no big deal. Sometimes I used food instead. I added 30 lbs of "entitlement" and I had a physical craving to sugar, you know after replacing 5 pints of vodka a day, I had the typical five stages of grief.

Q. Rebecca: And how do you feel today?

A. Travis: Today I feel completely blessed, extremely happy, never felt better.

Q. Rebecca: What do you do when someone offers you a drink?

A. Travis: It is usually at a work event for me when that happens, so that means it falls during the week and so I always say, "I don't drink during the week." And that is because I don't want to be judged for anything or be associated with anything about being a recovered alcoholic or something, in a work setting. But most circles that I have now know that I just live sober.

Interview #3
Laura

Q. Rebecca: When did you decide to quit drinking alcohol?

A. Laura: I thought about the decision to quit in September of 2008. But my official quit date is November 26th, 2008.

Q. Rebecca: Why did you decide to quit drinking alcohol?

A. Laura: I had gotten pregnant in a drunken blackout. It was the lowest I was ever willing to go. The lowest moral bar I had ever known in my life. I felt completely not in control of my life. I saw that I was having compulsive behavior.

So I started praying to the God of my understanding after I felt I wanted to quit. Then, I had a moment of clarity. I decided to quit on a day when I had been drinking all night long the night before. I was in the front yard of a friend's apartment in the morning. I came out of a black out and saw the sun coming through the trees. It was as though I had a moment of sobriety, a moment of clarity. And I heard a voice, it made me come out of the black out, and it said over and over, "you don't have to live this way anymore. Enough." Then I met my husband who was also recovering.

Q. Rebecca: Um, wow. This is now the third interview I have done. Not one of the people I had planned to talk to, did I know were alcoholics or addicts of any kind. I just thought I was going to be interviewing people who chose to not drink due to a healthy life style. I am actually about to drop my notes here because I am covered with goose bumps, chills and am freaking out a little. All three people have told me a very similar story, I mean almost verbatim. And maybe this is a typical alcoholic's experience when they do hit a rock bottom-type point in their life, but I have no idea. I had no idea! This is completely amazing. Just blowing my mind. I am sorry. Let's keep going. Ok, so how did you immediately feel after you decided to quit drinking?

A. Laura: Well I never went to treatment. I just dove into nutrition, organics, low carb, fitness, etc. I felt alive for the first time in my life, truly. More motivated, sleeping better, lost 30lbs. I felt so sick for so long, I just wanted to focus on being nice to my body.

But emotions would take over and I would cry sometimes, I had these moments. I had a supportive mentor at work who helped me through when I had these crying moments.

My entire life changed. When I was 9 months sober, an addiction center offered me a job helping other people get sober. It was incredible because the decision to quit drinking shifted me onto my life path. I could not have had one without the other.

Q. Rebecca: This is awesome stuff. So, how do you feel today?

A. Laura: It is 4 years today now I have been sober. I feel amazing. I have a responsible life, a disciplined life, crazy freedom, blessed life, health, balance, healthy friends. I love my job, it is the biggest no-profit treatment addiction center. (Laura works for Caron Treatment Centers)

Q. Rebecca: How do you handle social situations now when there is alcohol?

A. Laura: I ask for sparkling water when there is Champagne. I find it is actually more fun in social setting because I am present and engaged in.

When I am offered a drink, I just say, "no thanks" and it never goes beyond that. It is actually not that big of a deal ever.

Author's note: These first three interviews became the back bone of this book and also of my own sobriety. I had quit drinking a few weeks, maybe a month before these interviews happened. I am now typing today nearing my 90 day sobriety mark. What was a sober quest that I was just toying with, turned into a lifestyle and then a movement, a promise to myself and the world. I truly felt as though God was speaking to me and through these people. The remaining interviews are quite different and fall at the end of the book.

Chapter 3
HOW TO LIVE AN EXCITING, MIND BLOWING & FABULOUS LIFE

Q: My name is Aditi Ramchandani. I am the interviewer.

A. Rebecca: My name is Rebecca Sweeney. I am the Author.

Q: Please introduce yourself.

A. Rebecca: Hello, my name is Rebecca, and I am wellness and business coach. I help Moms and/or thirty something's who are depressed or want to be leaders and who want to have more inspiration and balance in their life. We focus on building better health, wellness, weight loss or weight balance, more happiness, success and joy. The direction we take is namely through sobriety, fitness, meditation and whole food nutrition.

Q: What will your target audience discover by reading this book?

A. Rebecca: My target audience will discover how to live consciously, absolutely live their most exciting and best life with things happening or starting to happen to them that they never even imagined, in the best ways through health and vitality, fitness, nutrition, sobriety and wellness.

Q: How does someone enjoy life in the most exciting, extraordinary way, in your opinion?

A. Rebecca: In my opinion, I have learned through my own experience, that the way to get the most nutrient rich and succulent experience in life is to be completely alcohol free but that combined with focusing on your own relaxation, fitness and nutrition, work and spirituality to bring a whole sense of being to your body, to your person, into your life; so that you can be fully present in your every experience that you go through.

Q: What do you find in common with people and addicts who have decided to quit drinking?

A. Rebecca: The interesting thing that happened to me when I decided to sit down and write a book, -it was suggested by a mentor to write a book about what I coach people on every day; and what I talk to people every day about are basically their frustrations and why they can't lose weight no matter what they do, no matter what they have tried and how they follow all these strict diet and exercise rules, why they're struggling with diet or nutrition; what their struggles are in life through fitness and health, and wellness in their body. But it always ends up translating into a deeper conversation. It's not just about how many sit-ups they do or how long they have exercised that week or how many calories they count; it always, always goes deeper than that.

So as a fitness coach I have gone on this journey myself. I was overweight, almost 60lbs or more overweight at one point, then had to battle with my own addictions through food and toxic substances, including alcohol. I started to focus on just fitness as a personal decision, I wanted to get into the best shape of my life when I was feeling somewhat depressed and in a rut of my own, in my early thirties. Just before I turned 30 was a really, really dark time for me.

And so I decided to focus on fitness and right around that time I got this gut feeling that I should just say goodbye to alcohol. I didn't necessarily categorize myself as an alcoholic. I am not a big fan of labels anyway. But I didn't know for sure or think that I really had a problem of any sort with alcohol, but I felt as though…when I thought of an author who I loved dearly, Dr. Christiane Northrup, I consider her just a beacon of light in women's health matters, especially health and wellbeing. I have at least two of her books. And a quote or two of hers, always stayed with me, in reference to how we do not listen to the sounds and signals of our body, "A dead giveaway that you are overextending, rather than stretching yourself, is the inability to nurture yourself or rest without a drink, a smoke, or overeating." In her book *Women's Bodies, Women's Wisdom,* she goes onto state how "Fifty percent of the accident victims in most emergency rooms are there because of alcohol abuse. As one of our staff anesthesiologists once said, 'If it weren't for cigarettes and alcohol, I'd be out of a job!" The entire first part of that book discusses the way we process pain, life and coping skills, or lack thereof. It all stuck with me for years and years.

We should not drink for that reason and we always have to find the relaxation within ourselves and with our own body's tools. To seek relaxation, you shouldn't be leaning on that drink. And that idea combined with several other things that have happened to me in my life, or people I have spoken with, just really, really stuck with me.

People who I really looked up to or respected, who never drank or had given up alcohol themselves, always stayed in the back of my head. And I felt like as I was going through my weight loss process I was getting a hold of every single thing in my life and empowering myself in every single way, but I never just decided to give up that alcohol because again, I didn't label myself as an alcoholic. I never had that "rock bottom" moment. So I felt like, if there's no problem then why should I let this go?

I had this gut feeling; it was like a far, far away feeling where I felt like I needed to quit and do it because of those reasons, of the people who I looked up to, who I honor and respected, who didn't have that as part of their life. And there had to be a reason for it.

So when I was sitting down after I'd achieved almost all of my weight loss, health and well-being goals, business goals, success in life, personally of my own as well as being a proud Mom of two: I was at a place where I was sitting down to write a book originally, I had not yet even given up alcohol.

However, that nagging feeling of wanting to do so was getting louder and louder and louder. So, when the interview process started with this book, I started to embrace a sober life. I was interviewing sober people and I literally felt like God was talking to me, through people, every single day. It was an amazing transformation for me, inwardly.

The people who I interviewed both at the beginning and the end of the writing of the book, totally shocked me and I had more than one moment of pure Divine intervention, is really the only way I could say it, because there was something that was occurring during these interviews that connected exactly perfectly verbatim to each and every interview. It shifted the way and the direction this book was going, and they all said something in the exact same way. These three people not connected whatsoever when they had given up alcohol, all said the very same thing in regards to why they gave up the alcohol and like it just ripped the rug from underneath my feet and completely blew me away. I knew *something* was happening in my life. And I loved it.

Q: Why do people quit drinking, for example, the people you know and interviewed?

A. Rebecca: Right, well the reason they quit was for health and wellness purposes, that's what I thought. So I learned that I quit drinking for a very different reason than the first stories in the book. But what was my Divine experience was, was the coincidence in the words used in my interviewees for this book. I mean it gives me chills just talking about it or thinking about it; I want to start to cry! Here's their story:

Each person, I keep reiterating that these people did not know each other at the time that they each had their experience, completely separate situations; different paths. Each person who I interviewed in the beginning, all said that they gotten to a place in their life where they were really drunk or just smashed or wasted or strung out on drugs, or something, at a point when it was almost as though their bodies or life situations could almost simply not handle it anymore. Their own rock bottom was a culmination of events and life choices leading up to what seemed a really pivotal and obvious moment to quit.

In this drunken or drug-stricken moment, they had a moment of sobriety, every one of the people said "I had a moment of sobriety" in the middle of my black out or drunken stupor. One friend was driving drunk and woke up in the middle of his blurry driving and thought to himself, "this would be my, (I think) third DUI (he said), and if I get another one that's a criminal record that I can't take away and I won't be able to drive or work anymore, and you've got to get your life together." He had a moment of sobriety and felt like he had a second where it was as though he heard a voice or God speak to him and just said all he could hear over and over and over again was "enough, no more of this, enough. This is enough."

He kept saying the word "enough" during that part of the interview.

When I heard everyone say that same thing, I started to feel something outside of me, separate from me, a force stronger than me, taking over my life, take over my direction, *my* sobriety.

By the third interview I was starting to cry and nearly dropping my phone in complete shock. I was not expecting these responses and not at all expecting the similarities.

I did not think I was going to be interviewing addicts who either wanted to go to rehab or needed to go to rehab. I didn't know that beforehand. I thought I just had these several people in my life who I knew of who decided to not drink and I wanted to know why, so I interviewed them.

One of the guys said I can recommend a few more people who were former alcoholics who would be happy to share their story with you, because most people like to talk about it. Most people who've given up drinking know exactly the day and will never forget it the rest of their life. They will shout out the date to you that they quit. It is like the celebration for them; it almost is like a birthday. This process in the book and in my life became this incredible chain reaction that opened up like a gorgeous flower.

It's actually like a rebirth to alcoholics who quit drinking. A lot of people think that it's such an awful thought to have to give up alcohol. It's almost as though I'm saying you can no longer have your birthday cake, or ice-cream or something really great in your life that you consider a part of celebration. Taking that away from you and how awful it is going to be, is an idea you can forget.

These people all proved and said it was like their life was more amazing than ever before, starting that day that they gave it up. Their lives keep getting better and better each year that progresses.

And you know of course there are hard days for us all but, it was so motivational and amazing and like a moment of speaking with God I really felt like Divine intervention in my life, again; that I was so moved by it that I felt that I needed to start a movement and I want to challenge and inspire people everywhere who both are alcoholics and have addiction problems and also with people who don't, more importantly!

I wanted to challenge people who don't have a problem with alcohol or who have NOT hit rock bottom yet, to hear these stories, consider joining us in this like, serious movement of clean and present living; be able to live fully present in their life. Each of the people sounded pure, yet actually drunk with happiness! To me, this was the most fabulous way to live. On a side note, nearly every single one of the sober people I interviewed has extreme success in their marriage and/or work, just blissful.

Q.: And could you go a little bit deeper into why you specifically stopped drinking? I know you started to touch upon it but if you could go a little deeper on that?

A. Rebecca: So I had that gut feeling for so long and I had those people in my life who I had looked up to, who none of them drank alcohol, and I will just go ahead and admit now, that I do believe I had a problem in some sense, and I'm going to go ahead and say that I think a lot of people who think they don't, actually do. Because I could never just stop at one glass of wine; I absolutely loved wine. And I don't think that is shameful to admit. Alcohol takes us over, when consumed, that is part of the lure, the 'letting go' feeling. The ritual takes us over, repeatedly, night after night, occasion after occasion. And so then it is a brain and life under the influence. It is not YOU making any more of your decisions, even if you don't drink all that often, it is you/your life PLUS this substance. I have no idea who the people are who have even just a little alcohol and still can manage to make completely clear, and good decisions in that moment of their drinking.

My drink of choice before a quit drinking, in my later life, was wine, as I have said. I absolutely loved wine. I used to think wine was just a delicacy, something so fine and elegant and it really wasn't. Well, to me it really wasn't. You know when I drank it, it lead me to more drinks and it lead me to money spending and my husband spending money, and buying more people drinks and really just sloth and just swollen joints the next morning, headaches, not sleeping well.

Even if I didn't have a full-fledged nauseous hangover it was still like you know, feel like crap the next day, even if you've had only a couple of glasses; especially if you go nine months without having any wine when you have a baby. I've had two babies and when you go back to drinking after pregnancy, I mean you just feel awful. It doesn't serve your body and yet you still do it and you drink and drink until you don't feel so awful and you get used to it again because you are dying for that sweet escape once more.

You know as you age, if I'm talking to people who are younger who might be reading this at some point, in my experience, as you age it gets less and less fun. I mean I'm not joking at all, it really does get less and less fun and it feels less and less good. When you wake up in the morning the hangovers are worse.

And the number one reason that I gave up drinking was not because I ever got to the point of those rock bottom moments like the people I interviewed who had a moment of clarity, I never experienced that. I had a soft quiet gut feeling for many, many years that I should do this and should make this choice as a Mom, a team leader, as a fitness coach, and for myself; and to just stop abusing myself because I associated every holiday, every wedding with alcohol.

I associated every celebration, every vacation this way. I just felt like, should vacation be a bunch of partying nights where you wake up feeling like crap the next day and it's ruined your whole next morning? No! Vacations should not be that, vacations should be restorative to our lives. And instead you have to recover from it most times 'cause people go and they "celebrate." And I wanted to start a movement with my own personal choice in my own life of: let's all take a look at how we celebrate and let's all take a look at how we can do it better and differently. You want world peace? You want better foods offered to us? You want better government leaders, or this or that in the world? START WITH YOURSELF, how about? Clean up your own life! Then it might spread, be a healthy trend, like this movement and we can collectively clean up the world!

People in India I think are the best example of celebration. I mean weddings last 10 days or more and they sing and they dance in Hinduism. You know there's not a lot of churches in America that have you dancing around and clapping. There should be more music and dancing, concerts offered with no substances around or for sale.

I think that we should also celebrate in a restorative, healthy, celebratory way and we're all just at Thanksgiving pouring alcohol, and Christmas, drinking at Christmas parties. And I just think that that doesn't feel good any more. It used to feel good when I was a lot younger. It used to be fun and wild and crazy and free and rebellious; and for some folks, those are all good feelings when you're young. But as you get older all of it stopped feeling good for me.

In fact there would be many, many nights, I would say nine out of ten nights when I decided to drink - girls night out or you know an art gallery show opening, or some special event (that should be special) I chose to take an alcoholic beverage which would always lead to like four or ten and I end up feeling horrible. I didn't feel drunk anymore. Celebration started feeling bad or sluggish or not good or celebratory as time went on. This was a huge motivator for me and is what keeps me sober.

When I got into my 30's I didn't get that drunk buzz, yah, happy feeling when I drank. I just felt sort of washed out, super bloated and chubby. I could drink ten drinks and not feel drunk, and not feel happy and not feel goofy. I would feel heavy, sugary and tired. Honestly, I don't know if it's 'cause I'm Irish, I have you know Irish blood and I have a tolerance of like a linebacker? I could just keep drinking, drinking, drinking and nothing good would ever come of it. And so from the fitness side of me and the weight loss side of me was like why, literally why, am I pouring all of these calories into my body? Why I am overdoing something that totally goes against my mission in life?

So that was my reason for giving up; that was my reason, alcohol no longer served me or my mission in life. It originally had nothing in common with the first three people who I interviewed who inspired me.

Q: By the way I am Hindu so I can vouch for all the dancing and stuff.

A. Rebecca: Yes! I love that, I love it!

Q: So how have you felt since you decided to quit?

A. Rebecca: The majority of the time has been the most comfortable and cozy, fuzzy, warm, lean, clean feeling, happy, relaxation and health and wellness and vitality I've ever felt in my whole entire life.

I won't lie and say that every single day has been that way. I won't lie and say I don't ever lose my temper with my children anymore. I won't say that I've lost 20 pounds (which I totally expected to)- that last 10 pounds I still want to get off, is still here. I won't say all those things have happened, it's not like a magic shift in my life in those ways, but what I do feel is that since quitting alcohol the workouts that I was doing before I quit alcohol, the same as I do now, are far, far more effective in less time.

You know I don't see my biceps get huge and cut and my gut lean in say, two days versus 20, as an example. No, it's not like that. I feel a good jump in my workouts like I'm getting a little bit further ahead than I was before because of this clean edge that I have of detoxification as a way of life, not just as a cleanse that we do every now and again but all the time I'm detoxified. And that is incredible, amazing, to live that way.

I do have more patience than I used to have with my children and- I don't know about my husband- but definitely with my children (laugh). No I have more patience than ever and that was always a problem for me. In traffic more patience - patience, patience, patience. I'm not perfect you know, like I said but I do see a drastic improvement.

I sleep better and I have more natural energy. Before you know I did the whole thing that most people do, I drank coffee in excess, like two cups a day, to wake up in the morning and I drank wine in excess to relax at night; and it was that vicious cycle that played into each other. I don't have that anymore and I like that a lot.

Q: You don't drink coffee anymore either?

A. Rebecca: I try not to. I still adore coffee. I still drink it. I try my hardest not to drink it every single day 'cause I don't like having addictions or feeling dependent on something or anything. And when I drink coffee everyday if I miss a day I get a headache and I get irritable and I don't feel good. Also, if I do drink it every day, that KICK that you get from it, no longer happens. To me that's an addiction, an addictive substance, and so I recommend not using it every single day and so I try to emulate that in my life. And like alcohol, coffee is extremely acidic to our insides and we need to learn about how damaging that can be over time to our inner health and balance of the body. We have to learn it is NOT just about how we look on the outside, that is a byproduct of wonderful inner balance and inner health.

I do fall into the trap of getting habitual with it and therefore I have to step back and look at it because I think we all have good habits and bad habits and I consider coffee a crutch that is not necessarily a good habit. I don't know if I'd call it a bad, bad habit; but I don't think it's a good one for sure. So no I don't drink it every day, just every once in a while.

Q: Does your husband often not drink?

A, Rebecca: No, my husband drinks every single day. That could be another reason, for all of this. He drinks beer. He is not a babbling drunk, who scares me or stumbles around. I have never heard his speech slurred. But most people are not that way, actually. He just depends on that beer at the end of the day to relax or to chill out or for his work day to decompress.

Q: That'd be something that I'd feel like me as your target audience would be interested in how that works.

A, Rebecca: Yeah I also didn't know if that was important to share or not, but I hope to be a leader and a good representation - what's the word I'm looking for - a good influence in my children's lives, as well as to my husband, and well as my team of fitness clients, in my fitness team of coaches and in my coaching. I am trying to represent what I feel is the way that I think that not necessarily the way that everybody should be but, I just want to be a good influence to everyone around me, authentic to myself, my role and my life, let's put it that way.

He is another human being, outside of myself, who makes his own choices. I have had opinions of him and other partner's choices before. And it does very little to concern yourself with what others do. Even a spouse. I honor whatever his path is. Do I wish he were sober? Sure. But I also know I would not have quit before it was my time if someone else just TOLD me to. So I don't concern myself too much with what he does in that area. It does not affect my life, really in any way. So I just focus on the positives.

Q: For example I'm your target audience and I'm considering trying what you're doing but I'm concerned about how this may affect my partnership, my marriage, because my partner drinks. So how do you deal with that or how does that play out in your life?

A, Rebecca: I don't ever believe anybody should quit drinking because somebody else wants them to, so I believe it should be a personal choice for everyone. I, believe it should be a choice if you know in your gut, like I knew in my gut, that it might be something that would really benefit you or be something really impactful to omit from your life. But I do know that most people who are sober, have partners who are sober as well. But not always. So it is not impossible to live in peace.

Because of all the reasons that I'm about to explain in the book, then it should be your choice. I don't believe you should make the choice for any other reason outside of yourself, but if you are worried about what other people around you think, how it will be with like your family, or your spouse, or your mate, or your partner, or your friends I suggest just trying it and seeing what would happen.

Because what most people think about what you drink, or what is going to happen when they stop drinking, -and I know this because I've interviewed people about it and I have done it, it's my own experience, I can tell you, it is SO not as big of a deal as you think it's going to be. It really doesn't matter. If one person drinks and the other does not, it really is our own personal choices and we just need to be with who we want to be with. If it is hard for you to resist alcohol with other people around you drinking, then you will have a hard time living this exemplary life. Just see it as, a choice you are trying for, living fully present, aware, clean, in the moment and not judging those around you for where they are in their path with alcohol.

Like when you go to a party it's awesome because you can drive home and you can drive whoever you're with home. And one reason I don't recommend AA and neither did one of the people I interviewed was because he felt like it was so limiting, 'cause they tell you not to hang out with people who drink; well that's like most people. At least 50% of the people in the world, drink.

Q: Yeah, that's interesting; I didn't know that.

A, Rebecca: That is almost impossible. So I recommend finding a way to hang out with people still who do. Now do I enjoy hanging out with people who absolutely love to drink and think it's just the coolest thing in the world and like want to get wasted every night? No. Those people don't inspire me anymore. Those are the people I hung out with for 30 years, up until I turned 30. Those were my friends. Those were the people, you know, everybody I worked with. That was everything I ever knew. I lived in a town that was very much like Mardi Gras every single night and had an "open container law" where you could leave work, meet a buddy at a restaurant or a bar, get a drink and stroll to the next bar with your drink in your hand; it was a drinking culture and my bosses did it and local government officials did it, among other horrific substances, and it was normal. It was what I thought was normal and you know getting out of that and turning your face towards a different option is really all about you; it really has nothing to do with anybody else, so don't let it.

So I'm here to tell you and repeat that if you're worried about, or concerned about how it's going to fit with other people: it really isn't that big of a deal, like it doesn't matter that much. And you know like I was going to take my husband out for his birthday tonight and we cancelled 'cause he wasn't feeling up to it, but I had thought about it and he was going to drink and I was going to drive and we were going to still celebrate. I would do it in my own way being fully present. And the people around me, I would let them do it in their way and their process and not judge them either. And I thought about it beforehand and I was good with it all. I set an intention.

But I choose, as a personal choice, I choose for me and choose respect for others, no matter what. I choose to hang out with and I really respect people who have made the choice to not have alcohol in their life for various different reasons. But I don't ever judge people who do drink; I don't. I used to be a drinker. I'm just now here to offer another perspective.

Q: What's the longest you've gone without drinking?

A. Rebecca: So before now, I'm speaking to you today, what is the date today, the 20th of April, 2013 and I have only been sober, one hundred percent clean and sober for a little over two months. But I went over a year without drinking when I was pregnant and had a baby and wanted to be a nursing mom, who was super clean for a few months post-delivery. But with both children I don't really consider that authentically sober… making the choice not to drink for a baby is not making a choice to not drink for yourself; its protecting something else. So it has nothing to do with the personal choice, in my opinion.

So I can say that I mean its pretty joyful for me right now to say that I think that this is the first time I've made the choice for myself completely, and it's the longest I've ever gone in that decision, since I was like 14 years old.

Q: Who or what books motivated you to quit drinking?

A. Rebecca: What books?

Q: Any people and any books?

A. Rebecca: I'm going to start with the people. Tony Horton, the fitness genius, inspired me to live this way because I had heard him on the Dr. Oz show say once, "I don't drink alcohol or caffeine." It resonated with me. But the first person who ever motivated me or sparked an interest in my brain to not drink was an exemplary guy named Anis Mojgani and he was a friend of mine in college and he was of the Baha'i Faith. He told me in our second year of college that he's never had a sip of alcohol in his entire life - he was older than me too - and he never planned to drink. I said why, I asked him about that once and said why, you know like, what in the world? Never?

And he said because in my faith, in my religion we are taught not to drink alcohol and so I don't. And it was as simple as that. And I said why, why do they do that in your religion? And he then said one thing that always stuck with me and still to this day does and always has, and it's been well over 15 years since he said this to me, he just looked at me and he said because,

"alcohol rots your brain."

-period.

I mean it does nothing for you, health-wise and the people will argue that you know a drink or a wine, one glass here and there or once a day is good for your heart, -bull, I say. I can give you ten other things in my opinion that are better for your heart and your blood pressure than drinking that alcoholic beverage, and for example going for a brisk walk. I really don't think your cardiovascular health needs to depend on alcohol, so that's not an excuse in my mind, or a reason.

The other person is who I mentioned, Dr. Christiane Northrup, she made that quote I referenced earlier about why you go to drink that drink. Most people, even healthy people who are not considered alcoholics will say, "I am so stressed out right now, this is why I need a glass of wine, or this is why I need a beer, or this is why I need that, or I deserve this drink." It's not the right reason and its preventing your body in my opinion from utilizing the God-given intuition and problem solving skills that we have; it's hiding that, its depleting that, it's numbing and ruining that skill set, slowly over time. It is so different from saying, "I deserve this piece of wedding cake, or this ice cream treat." Because treats do not alter your state of thinking and being like alcohol does. Soon you're not going to have that choice any more to utilize your skills that are naturally born in your body - fight or flight chemicals that we have will be numbed, if you constantly go to that alcoholic beverage instead of utilizing your own body's systems to get you through hard times or whatever you struggle with, your neurons will not fire correctly when stress arises, if alcohol is not there to get you through it.

So Dr. Northrup and all of her books on the body and our inner wisdom are awesome in that subject matter. One of the other people that I always looked up to - I used to work for a nutrition company and my business partner and mentor there was a man named David McLaughlin (interview #1) and he always told me that he didn't drink, and I always thought he just made the personal choice to live a healthy, clean life, and I didn't realize that he had a really sticky history with abuse. He motivated me heavily to quit drinking. Actually almost all of the people who I interviewed motivated me to quit alcohol. And I could list more but I feel like I'm going on and on.

Q: Any one book that comes to your mind?

A.: Rebecca: One of Dr. Christiane Northrup's books, *Women's Bodies Women's Wisdom,* any of her books, as well as the *Slight Edge* by, Jeff Olson. I consider that book by Jeff Olson being a phenomenal book that you can translate into health and wellness because he talks about how it's not really one big decision that makes you healthy, that makes your life successful, it's a bunch of tiny, tiny, tiny little choices that are slight and miniscule that all add up to one big, amazing life. And that's how it is with drinking in my mind. It's not just the big decision to quit drinking, it's the miniscule tiny, little times when you're having a hard day and you want a drink; those moments, those tiny, little moments that you choose the brave choice and the smart choice in my mind, those are the ones that pay off big in the long run and end up yielding the HUGE results.

And so that book and all of my business as well as yoga books I sort of translate into health, sobriety and wellness even though he and the other authors relate their writing more from a business aspect or fitness, but you cannot enjoy all of these business or body benefits from a toxic place. You cannot. Those two listed above are the first that come to mind, but I have a long list of recommended texts I will list in the end of the book.

Q: And you mentioned how you felt after you decided to quit, I just wanted to ask you how those other people felt after they'd quit. Was it similar to yours, or was there anything else you wanted to add about how their experience was after they stopped drinking?

A. Rebecca: Everybody has said that they feel absolutely, incredible, fabulous and amazing. I was expecting them to feel like "-mmm, ehhh." Oh yeah that reminds me, just remembered! This is one of the books I also recommend. There's a book called *Smashed: Story of a Drunken Girlhood* by Koren Zailckas, that I read a long time ago which was another little sobriety seed planted in my brain, written by a young girl who was just sort of fed up and mortified with the way that people drink. And actually how American colleges abuse alcohol, basically how society abuses alcohol throughout growing up and into adulthood.

It's really sort of an epidemic to me, it's not anything to be taken lightly; how frat parties always equal getting wasted, and going to college and gaining "the freshman fifteen," that doesn't always come from poor food choices. I mean it's pretty scary and awful the drinking that goes on in college.

And this book *Smashed* goes over that and in that book she always talked about how she didn't really feel, when she made the choice to quit drinking, nothing great happened in her life after, she did not feel anything wonderful, but she just still stuck with her guns in that she didn't want to drink anymore.

I had the complete opposite experience and so did nearly everyone I interviewed. They all said life was amazing in one word, just incredible, beyond fabulous, and better than ever, after they'd quit.

CHAPTER 4
HOW TO LIVE WITH FABULOUS SUCCESS

Q: Why don't most people succeed in the health arena part of their life, or health-wise I guess you could say?

A. Rebecca: I feel like we are inundated with food choices that are not good for us. The majority of the choices that we're given for food are usually straight up *not* good and that's not our fault. We have to take it upon ourselves to educate ourselves. And that's annoying really, to be honest, because who has time to sit down and study nutrition when they've got busy lives and having to learn and scour: what are the ingredients in our food that are good for us and not good for us? I just think that's awful that we have to do that today, but we have to do that and that's one thing that's slowing down everyone's metabolism, is the amount of processed foods, chemicals and the lack of exercise, along with the cultural alcohol choices, substances, it is all of it combined together, in my opinion.

We have a very sedentary life in the modern world where we drive to work in a car sitting, we sit at a desk all day long, drive home sitting, and we sit on the couch and watch TV when we get home in the evening and then off to bed. It's all sitting, resting and that's why there's over 80 percent of the world has lower back problems now because we don't even use our backs correctly; we don't use our bodies right, how they were intended, or we really don't even use them at all.

And so I think that's also a main point, the sedentary lifestyle is like the second main point, after foods. And the third is obviously the common use and abuse of alcohol I believe, in our modern society.

Rebecca Sweeney

Q: Why do you feel like most people don't succeed in their finance and career?

A. Rebecca: I feel like most people should be entrepreneurs, that is what I think we are all really designed for and I feel like most people have it in them to be. I think God created us to be sort of like artisans of all different types, we should all barter and trade with each other because everybody has something to offer, every single person, in a unique way. Everyone has a gift. And I believe everyone should be paid nicely for it, so long as we recognize and utilize that gift or gifts.

And I just feel like nobody teaches people how to do that, how to work for themselves and that feeds into the fact that nobody feels their own personal power, or their inner wisdom, which feeds into the fact that we don't study and really take control of the foods that are going into our bodies, which feeds into the fact that we go along with the crowd and we drink whatever they drink, relax and cope how they cope and we do whatever they do and we just do what society does.

And the majority of society is not wildly successful because we just sort of are walking in circles together. And it's the wild, crazy people who break out and want to run their own business and don't have support from really anybody in their life, so it's the super wild and crazy brave people who actually make it a lot of the time, because they've had to usually do it all alone, out on their own with no support and no education in how to do it. And if they don't give up on their crazy dream they make it. But most people do give up, then they end up in the majority again. And I just feel like this all goes back to this circle of consumption; what we're fed, what we drink, what everyone else does anyway and so I think it's all part of each other, one reason America is the most obese country, etc. We drink the way everyone drinks around us and we eat the way the big, affordable stores sell to us and how everyone around us eats because we are numb to feel or think otherwise. Funny thing though, America is also one of the most amazing countries for STARTING your own business, so the ones who do and choose the right business model, have incredible amounts of personal success. Which I think should be celebrated and supported by everyone, much, much more.

I think finance balance, career balance, personal power balance, religious balance, relationship balance, that's all connected, so it's all part of each other and to be your own boss, you almost have to have all of this in play together, at once. So it is all connected. Not easy to do, not the easy road, surely. But SO worth it.

Q: What should people do if they want to become an entrepreneur?

A. Rebecca: So if they want to become an entrepreneur I recommend studying people like Paul Zane Pilzer, a world class economist, or Robert Kiyosaki, the author of *Rich Dad Poor Dad*, because they believe, they are these great financial leaders and they're very well trained and learned and educated in finance and money, spending, and profit and business models. I've been following their advice and watching their studies and practices for almost a decade now. And they love the network marketing model because it leaves it up to the person, the individual totally and one hundred percent.

The scary part about that is that people don't believe in themselves enough to do successful things with it. And the negative connotations that go along with it, like I'm going to be expected to sell to my mom and dad and my neighbor. And then third they don't know about it, like people aren't educated in entrepreneurial matters unless they go and take it upon themselves to learn, just like the food they are "fed" or otherwise, if they listen to somebody who wants to talk to them about it. It is hard to find solid, honest training and education on all of this so people are wary.

Another thing that Robert Kiyosaki says is that you have to think in opposites. It is an excellent success tip. If something is not working in your life what's the opposite that you should be doing? And he says something along the lines of, "I didn't ever want to pay taxes, I just didn't and so I did things to earn money that didn't involve taxes, like buying and selling stuff and making a profit where I didn't have to be taxed on it, and not 'working' in a job. I didn't want to get a job because my money would be taxed, so instead I learned how to sell stuff that was tax free, or saved money that was tax free." And so he just does as his rich dad taught him, the opposite of what everybody else would normally think to do. This translates to so much in our life to benefit us, -brilliant.

And I think you need to think that way in your life. Anytime you have a problem -think in oppositions. "Well I'm not getting what I want in my relationship," so maybe you're not *giving* that in your relationship. So instead of thinking of all of what you're not getting, you need to give. Give, give, give, be, be, be and then all of a sudden things will slowly but surely start to turn around.

And so I recommend reading books like '*The Secret*' and *The Power*, even though a lot of times these days people think that's all cliché, but if you just pound it into your brain over and over and over and self-educate and work for yourself anybody can start a network marketing company, and anybody- literally I'm not lying, I'm not being pie in the sky, *anybody* can be a millionaire and so you just have to do it, plan it and not only do it, **expect it**.

Q: What have you learned from network marketing?

A. Rebecca: So network marketing has been my greatest teacher because it's given me the confidence to go against the grain when like I said everybody in my life didn't support it or understand it and I did it anyway. It's not that they didn't really believe in me, it is just back to the fact that they didn't see me working for a "boss" so they didn't understand it, or understand how to support it, my business.

So it gave me all this strength that I'd never had and belief in myself that I didn't have. I had no self-esteem. I had very, very low self-esteem for most of my life and network marketing really challenges your courage, talking to people, looking people in the eye, approaching people, getting to know why you have certain fears.

Because if you don't do anything, if you stay in your little corner afraid in the dark, you're not going to make any money. And so if you step out of the dark and you do something that really scares you, (a) you learn from it personally, and (b) you sort of ask yourself why is this scary to me? And the answers are enlightening.

And so it's like a self-help life if you let it be. And so I think everybody should be in the network or relational marketing industry and so does Paul Zane Pilzer. He believes that is like the number one best thing to do; and on a side note he also believes that being in the wellness industry, as well as network marketing, is the best choice for everyone because the wellness industry isn't going anywhere. It is slowly but surely going to pass over the sickness industry; like he refers to it, which is pharmaceuticals, hospitals and that field - doctors, nurses, sickness. Prevention and health and wellness is where we are headed and where money is growing and where it's going to be forever because it's just the safest bet, both personally in your own life through your personal choices of food, alcohol, everything, as well as business. It's a smart, smart business choice. I recently got to hear him speak, which was a dream of mine for almost ten years. And he said, you have to remember, "would you like to spend a small fortune on a disease later? Or would like to spend smaller amounts **now** on your wellness?" (referring to the wellness and fitness products like my company sells)

Q: What have you learned from being your own boss versus being a manager?

A. Rebecca: When I was a manager, 'cause I've managed a major corporation's store, I was an assistant manager and also the head manager of a store once, I found I was more motivated to just get by and just do enough to not lose my job. I didn't realize then but I realize now looking back at it. I thought I was doing a phenomenal job back then and I think I did do a pretty good job as those positions go, but I realize now that I didn't have the get up and go that I have for my own business, because I was always going to get the same amount of money, no matter whether I tried really, really hard, or I barely tried at all. I might get a tiny promotion in a year or two. I might get to district manager for like $10-20,000 more *someday*. You know it was nothing motivational that really drove me or pushed me forward.

In being your own boss you can push, push, push for a week and rank advance and get substantially more money in a week and a half. You can go from making $3,000 a year to six figures in less than two years in network marketing. And on my team it literally happens all the time to people. It's pretty amazing. So the motivation and the do or die feeling of working for yourself kicks the ass off working for somebody else.

Another awesome part of finding your own financial success in this way, is that you can build it, your very own business, WHILE you are working for someone else's business (j-o-b). So it does not HAVE to be "do or die." It can be a slower progression of building for you. You are king there, and make those choices. And my team is always hiring! So contact me, seriously, to help you (laugh)!* I have a lot of coaches and business partners who celebrate their spouse retiring at age 32 when they make it big in their own business in like 14 months and fire their boss, or pay off their house. It really is the most delicious success. You just have to make sure you find a team to join and business that fits you well, which is totally achievable. But when you do, it is completely fabulous.

*E-mail me for the information regarding joining my team at: Rebecca@taohappiness.com

CHAPTER 5
HOW TO LOOK FABULOUS

Q: Interesting! Back to talking about the weight loss. How did you feel before you lost a good amount of weight?

A. Rebecca: Well the reason that I wanted to get fit and do all these things in my life that I've done towards wellness was in large part because I have a lower back condition called Lordosis -which in my research of Lordosis, and experience with people in fitness in general, I think that a lot of people have some form of it more than they know, and if they weren't born with it like I think I was, they develop it through a weak belly or a fat belly. It makes your lower back curve in excessively and it causes a lot of pain; so a lot like I said before over 80 percent of the people in the world have lower back pain. Lordosis is also called swayback.

So I lived with chronic pain. I was so overweight. I will be honest and say, I don't like to talk about it but, I was a smoker at one time. I was always a closet smoker, on again and off again all my life. Everyone around me in school did it, so I followed along, more "sheep" activity there. Then when I had children (I never smoked while pregnant or nursing), after they were big enough to know, I would try to hide it from my kids. I was just thinking after a while, I'm simply not going to do this. I'm not going to have kids who know that I smoke and I'm not going to be hiding from them either. A lot of other people in my life I was comfortable hiding from for some reason, but I was never going to hide from my kids.

So when my oldest daughter got older I just thought, no more smoking and that lead me to just being like I'm not going to be in this fat, painful, body any more either,

I'm too young and have too much life to live to see how horrible I'm going to feel and how this can only get worse and worse and worse as I get older. So I was depressed, angry, short tempered, very unattractive and just a horrible model as a human being and I was wasting away and feeling pretty crappy.

And all the while I was feeling all of those things, I was a yoga instructor too, can you imagine? So I just knew, I'm just not even a product of the product, like I just need to get my stuff in order. I was not practicing what I was preaching. So I was pretty miserable all the way around. I always felt like a damaged fraud.

Q: How much weight have you lost?

A. Rebecca: Today I have lost a total of 40-50 pounds and I'm shooting to reach a 60 pound weight loss; between a 50 and 60 pound weight loss -I would say, I will know it when I feel it.

Q: How did you get in shape? What was your start?

A. Rebecca: Well this is what I want everyone to know, is that it is a process and it doesn't have to be like ripping a band aid off, or: I'm going to take your coffee, your bread, and your alcohol away all in day one of boot camp. What I did, I suggest other people do, is I changed nothing about my diet and my alcohol intake. All I did was get off my butt, off the couch and start moving and did a fitness program. This is what gave me my beauty back. My light. The light that everyone has, vitality. It leads you to better and better and better decisions which all bring natural and radiant beauty and health out from deep inside. Beauty that no one ever probably knew they had, or ever tapped into. -So long as you don't give up on the process.

That is one of the tricks. When you get started slowly, just make sure you know that this is a new life style. This movement, as slow as it is going to start, is going to be something that you do for the rest of your life. It will evolve, it might not always look the same, but it is something that you will be doing forever. So commit, get used to the idea and never, never, never give up on yourself. "Never, never, never give up," like Winston Churchill said.

Of course I'm going to plug my company; I became a part of my company because of how much I loved it and I'm going to plug it like shamelessly in my book because I love it so much, but the first program in getting my butt in gear was P90X from Beachbody. It turned my life around because it gave me a specific schedule that was very easy to follow, easier than a personal trainer at a gym would give, and I had a whole entire community of people who were so positive and amazing and like a prayer answered in my life, people who cared and were rooting for me came out of the woodwork; all the people affiliated with the company and my personal coach and our team that just right away came with it. It was really an incredible community and decision.

So I lost 20 pounds in three months just from doing this workout and then the magical thing about our body and fitness is that when you start moving your body just naturally, it's the law of attraction, the snowball effect, whatever you want to call it, the body just naturally wants more and more things that are good. It tells you that it wants better food, you crave salad more, it's very simple, it's nothing crazy or woo-woo or super out there, it's just very basic natural science. THIS is mind-body. You crave more things, you crave better things, you take care of your body, your brain follows suit. You take care of your brain, your body follows suit. It's just like the feeling of thirst that you get when you're dehydrated; your body tells you what it wants and then also you hear it better when you're healthier and you are focusing more *on* your body.

You become more and more and more and more in tune to what is good and what is right. And you just have to know the tricky part is that the healthier and healthier you get, you just have to listen. Sometimes we don't want to listen to what our body is actually telling us and so we have to learn to really listen to the subtle sounds and noises and signals of the body-not the brain. The brain is trained to do everything you have done *up* until this point in your life today. The intuition, the body, the will is what you listen to, to change that brain and move it into a better way of thinking and being.

And so then the next step of the process was that I changed my diet. I wanted better results, I wanted to look better, I wanted to feel better; I was liking what I was seeing and I wanted more. So then I realized okay I've got to stop eating chocolate chip cookies and cheese crackers all day and I've got to clean up my nutrition a little bit more. And so I did go and study, that was a natural progression, studying more about like all the different ways you can eat, fuel and nourish your body through food. And then it lead me to a super, super clean choice (after about two years of this fitness focus) of limiting then a hundred percent omitting, the alcohol. And so it was a natural progression that was slow for me, it wasn't like ripping a band aid off.

Q: That's fascinating. How does one maintain after a huge weight loss?

A. Rebecca: So that is the most important thing I want people to know as well, is that a lot of times people will look at a really intense workout program that seems so hard and so intense, intimidating and so many hours, and that might be something that certain people need to get into shape. But unless you're like an Olympic trainer or bodybuilder of some sort in competition, the important thing I want everyone to know, is that you do not have to continue; once you've reached most of your goals in fitness and weight loss and nutrition and health, you don't have to keep beating yourself into that workout to maintain it.

Once you've achieved and worked hard through the initial tougher parts of conditioning an out of shape body, all you have to do is light maintenance, two to three, four days a week, 20, 30 40 minutes. It's not as intense as the getting there. That is so important to know and remember! So once you've gotten there you've got this sweet ride for the rest of your life that maintaining is so much easier, and enjoyable, than getting 50 pounds off, or 100 pounds off, or whatever it is for each person.

Q: Can you speak more on why wellness is the best industry to be in right now?

A. Rebecca: I already answered that one too in my previous blab, going on about Paul Zane Pilzer; because it is trending in all different sorts of statistical graphs to slowly be beating out the pharmaceutical industry to sum it up. The pharmaceutical industry is what fixes people when they're sick and in my opinion is what wants to keep people down and on the drug that they provide and they sell. So why would they ever create a pill that makes you well that you don't have to take anymore? Cause then they would be out of business.

So it's not a smart industry to be in, the sickness industry. The best industry to be in is the wellness industry because it's not a bad thing, it's not a fad, it is not scam, it makes your back or injuries feel better, you know, people always need to stay in shape, they always need to give that gift to their body every single day. So any fitness related or wellness related job is the smartest economically for you, for the future. It's never going anywhere, it's never going to change in technology and the more we learn about it the better the industry becomes financially. People are supposed to be projected to spend more money on prevention than on illness in the near future and so you know, I think people should stick with that financially as well as just dive into it! Get into fitness! Get into wellness! For your financial health and physical health! It is a win-win.

Q: What if I had no support in sobriety or the wellness business? How do I maintain and keep strong?

A. Rebecca: Right, it's the same thing that I've been talking about. I didn't have any support in sobriety either. I didn't have any support in my fitness; my kids were young, it was hard to find time to work out. My husband he was supportive with my business just somewhat and my fitness but he doesn't really work out with me very much. He is busy, in the military, we live a busy, moving stressful life, all the odds were against me. That is how I chose the fat, drown my sorrows, drink wine on couch-road.

And a lot of people who I coach say that their husbands or their spouses or their friends will even make fun of them if they focus on healthy eating or diet, because they're coming from a place probably of unhealthiness or fear of their own wealth and health, so they feel threatened and will either make fun of or not support or shun people who are doing something really positive and healthy that they're excited about in business, entrepreneurially or health and wellness like I've talked about.

I think it's all connected as I've said and what you have to do is make your own choices no matter what. If you've got a spouse who says, "I refuse to eat that healthy crap," you make a separate plate for yourself and you don't cave in and eat the junk that they want to eat, and you be a beacon of light in people's lives. It's your responsibility for yourself and for all the people around you in my opinion. There is always going to be temptation, so don't feed your excuses or negative thinkers around you. Just go on your path and stand firm. Ignore the people who do not support you.

Q: Why do you promote always having a plan B if you suggest always staying positive?

A. Rebecca: So the point of this is, I don't agree with always "planning for the worst and hoping for the best." I don't like that statement or mind set at all. I feel like you should plan for the best and have a plan B, just in case, or should things shift, like life always does. I feel like you should just flip that perspective.

We shouldn't just plan for the best and think everything's going to be perfect. I mean I promote staying positive in every single thing you do; don't let anybody bring you down, like I was just talking about. But you know positivity, positivity, positivity should be your goal in several things that are happening in your life. If something "bad" is happening to you, in your relationship, in your health, think positive, find the blessing, find the lesson behind it. Positive thinking: it's very, very well known today that that's what gets you what you want... your perspective, it changes your mind then changes your life.

But life happens and there are usually very valid reasons that people come into struggles and so you should see that in a positive way, as a gift. Struggles teach us things; they control our lives and blessings sometimes, yea -even the struggles. And for example when we're talking about something as simple as a workout, let's say I have a plan to work out every single day at 6:00am, well what if my baby throws up that morning? I'm not going to be able to work out at that time because she's just gotten sick. So you have to have a plan B.

You have to have plan B if you are in business. If you are in business I say don't put all your eggs in one basket. Have several ways of making money. If you can't work out and that's the same example, if you can't work out at 6:00am like you planned, have a time where you know that's your second choice. Always have a second, sometimes third choice and stay positive about doing both, and knowing that you've always got a safety net but don't always, always plan for the worst, hope for the best-attitude. I just don't like that, I like it to flip the other way.

Q: How have your life choices lead you to sobriety, financial and spiritual balance?

A. Rebecca: I just want to say again, I don't judge anyone for drinking and I'm going to answer a question that I have often too: I don't believe in like outlawing alcohol or prohibition or anything like that. I think that our poor choices or our choices of unhealthy toxic things sometimes are what lead us to Divinity and to our higher self. And so I think that my wild, self-abusive past gave me the tools to be an even better leader today than I could have ever been, because if I didn't go through everything that I went through, made the stupid mistakes that I have made, how would I ever be able to understand all of the people who I coach on a daily basis, on my team and how would I ever know where they're coming from?

I feel like a little bit like the Chaka Khan song, like *I'm Every Woman,* hahah, I can connect with, all different types of women because I've done so many different things good and bad, and the bad ones I embrace too and I'm not afraid to share because it is what's going to help me connect with people. I believe everybody should live a very open life for that reason. Just like babies and children slip, fall, do naughty things, it is all their way of learning how to BE in this world, learning how to grow.

We need to just brush off our past errors, poor choices and devote ourselves to the fabulous, bright future that we are better now able to recognize. And this all comes together when we devote ourselves to fitness and improving our bodies.

Following prayer, devotion to my own self-righteousness, seeing myself as a child of God, made in God's image, focusing on goodness for myself, my marriage and my children, all of this has lead me out of my struggles and troubles and into my success. Also never giving up, even when things seem like hell on earth. No matter how much I have hated myself in the past for a myriad of reasons, I always had this Yogi's quote posted in my kitchen, where I walked every day: "Do good and be good and the entire wisdom will be yours." -Sri Swami Satchidananda. Searching for that good was my only plan.

CHAPTER 6
WHY ALCOHOL IS A LIFE NUMB-ER

Q: Why do people want to be numb? -Why do you call alcohol a life numb-er?

A. Rebecca: Why do people drink and why do people choose alcohol? I believe it's because they want to numb the sensations of life for two reasons. Because I think life causes pain and people don't want to feel the pain that comes along inevitably with life. And second, I believe that people, the statement that sometimes you hear where, people are afraid of their own success and their own power.

So why is that? I think the reason for that is because of the pressure that they think inevitably that will come when they step into their own power, like "oh how am I ever going to actually succeed once I get the success I know I want?" Or they just don't believe in themselves enough; I'm not good enough to do this thing that I know that I really am blessed enough to do, or maybe I won't be able to handle the responsibility of personal power or leadership, these are all thoughts and feelings we have deep inside.

They're afraid of their own strength and the responsibility that comes along with it, so I think that they keep everything away. Like they're afraid of pain and they're afraid of success and so I think they choose alcohol to escape from feeling the rawness of life. They choose to stay in a numb state and in the middle.

Q: What are people hiding from in their lives? Why do people not think they feel good enough while sober in life? Or why do they not feel good enough while they're sober?

A. Rebecca: I don't think people, on the whole, are never taught relaxation techniques or coping skills. We take an Advil when a headache comes instead of trying a healthy snack or glass of water first, maybe your body is telling you that you need more water or a nutrient? I don't think people are taught how to listen to their bodies, how to utilize intuition and so when they're sober they feel like they're missing out on something that alcohol can give, which is a looseness, a wildness, a freedom, relaxation that comes from perfect health, balance. That in sober life takes discipline to feel, but you can feel all those things, but they either don't want to put the time in to learn how (just like with our food intake choices), or they don't believe they can feel those things naturally.

Q: Why do people drink with little kids?

A. Rebecca: Oh I've heard this among my peers and people in my age group a lot, that it is so stressful to have this life where children are given to you after pregnancy and no one *really* teaches you how to be a good parent. I'm not sure why parents don't pass it down verbally to their children more on how to be a good parent because it's a lot like running your own business. Everyone says, "oh I cannot tell them how to parent, that's not my job." It's something that's not taught - so you're thrown into this thing that's wild and uncontrollable and completely confusing and scary. But people don't want to tell people how to parent, so we just stay silent and are left with the responsibility to look up parenting books and hope that we find one we like, if we find the time to read it among all the changing diapers, let's hope we can apply it!

They (parents) often don't know how to cope so they seek a very, very easy escape in alcohol and it's stressful and so they 'wanna get out and they can't get out so they're 'gonna like numb themselves just to get through it and I think it happens all the time. It happened to me!

Q: Why is sober parenting so important?

A. Rebecca: Well for the very simple reason that what if there's an emergency? I mean nobody ever talks about that. Shouldn't we want to have our best wits about us at all times as parents? What if your kid chokes in their sleep and you were too black out drunk to hear them? What if you need to drive them somewhere, I mean I guess you can call 911 but what if they just broke an arm and don't really need an ambulance but certainly need professional care? You would not call an ambulance for that. I just always think about what if you need to drive or answer quick, specific questions and you're sitting round with all your friends getting wasted and your kids are upstairs playing or sleeping. It is essentially leaving them unattended, in my mind.

I've done it and I used to think about that when I first had kids and I think people just accept it. But it is one place where you should NOT hope for the best, "oh well" attitude, but instead always be prepared for anything. It is completely numbing yourself off to responsibility and being present for that child or those children. I feel like alcohol is a legal drug and it's just something that completely skews your judgment and your parenting and I think it's important to be one hundred percent present in your children's life and hundred percent present to me means: **sober**. And not hung over, because I don't think people would beat their children as often if they were always sober, I don't think people would lose their temper as often and I think people would actually, by nature and without much effort, just teach their children then to find ways of coping that don't involve alcohol, just by example, not by words alone.

We (society) teach them to drink by example! Imagine what we would teach them by example, no other effort, if we did not drink alcohol? And so we're expanding the minds and potential of our future, our humanity by choosing sober parenting. And this is just by starting with ourselves.

Q: What do people miss out on when they're drinking alcohol?

A. Rebecca: What do people miss out on?

Q: Yes, like you said 'not being fully present for life'.

A. Rebecca: You miss out on everything, you miss out on usually the best occasions because like I said, when we celebrate we drink, when we dine out, we drink, so you're missing out on the very best moments of your life when you're drinking, to sum it up quite simply. It is you: on something, instead of absorbing everything. You might miss some bad stuff when you are under the influence, but more so, you are missing so much good stuff too.

Q: How do you tell people to handle the pain without alcohol?

A. Rebecca: So when we feel pain, whether it be physical pain or emotional pain, the best way that I have found is a sort of concentration technique to deal with pain: it's not to push it away and not to do the opposite, the positive, like say, "Oh thank you so much for this *blessing* and this pain." No.

When you're in the acute moment of dealing with the emotional or physical pain, the best thing that I have found in my personal experience is to close your eyes for a second or longer and say, "I'm not pushing it away and

I'm not grateful for it, I am just aware of it and I'm just sitting with it - I'm just accepting it, I'm just being present with this pain." And then you name it. You describe it, you come up with a way to explain it like you are explaining something to a four year old. For example, this pain is hot, sitting in the part of my neck below my skin, next to my shoulder and it tingles and feels sharp, etc. And nine times out of 10 it completely goes away or greatly eases when you start to do that, or those types of techniques: just accepting it and sitting with it, saying, "I sit with this pain, I sit with this thing that I'm feeling right now. I am just sitting with this struggle." Nothing more. It takes repition and practice. But, it just vanishes, it's like magic and I can go into more of that technique in the book, near the meditation section. And I have a free, pain dissolving meditation on my web site meditation page. www.taohappiness.com/meditation

Q: How do you tell people to handle fear without alcohol or would it be the same technique, or different?

A. Rebecca: Yes, I was taught many years ago, by a friend named Ornesha, that the best way to deal with fear is to think about your breath and through many breath work techniques that I teach and we touch on in this book. But just be very basic, start small, returning your mind to your breath, how it goes in, how it goes out and over and over and over and over, it does so many things: It brings you to the present moment, it reminds you that you're alive, it reminds you that you're a human being – have a God-given right of life, and it helps you deal with your fear.

It pushes away anything that could hurt you because your breath is your gift and it's usually involuntary (we don't think about it) but when you think about it all this world of light can come through breath work.

There is a man in India named Yog Sandesh who teaches yoga and basically he just teaches breath work and it is the tunnel way, the road to nirvana because there are so many ways just to focus on breath that can take you from your fear. That just shows the power of focusing on the breath. It is what a nurse would suggest when a patient feels anxiety, or a rapid heart rate due to stress. So I work with people in meditations that way.

Q: What happens when people are hung-over?

A. Rebecca: When you're hung-over you're missing out, you're doing more missing out and numbing only it is not half as fun as the night before. You are subtracting that time from your life what you could have been doing. So you subtracted the night before, your presence was gone when you were doing the drinking. And your life is barely present or not fully there when you are hung over the next morning. That is taking almost one full day from your life in total. So I consider drinking, I consider smoking, I consider all of the toxic things that you can do to your body through drugs or alcohol or poor food choices to be a very slow form of suicide. That's what my Dad always said about smoking and I have quoted him several times.

I had a counselor once, I would love to tell the story, I was in marital counseling and we brought up the topic of cigarettes and how I wished they weren't in my marriage anymore. I told her that I considered smoking a slow form of suicide, I had given it up, but my partner still smoked and I felt like you're choosing to hurt yourself when you smoke and she said, "Oh no, no, no, that's not what smoking is, people don't smoke for that reason."

But I disagree, I really do believe that deep, deep down inside - maybe it's even subconscious - it's a choice to hurt yourself and a hangover is the same: it's a choice to take away some part of your life. If you really, really think about it you don't want that, you want to have the best life you can have. You 'wanna get the most out of life and hangovers steal that. You are trading a very, very temporary buzz for a price of time loss and not feeling well. It seems simple. But we all must be in that much fear and pain, that we are willing to make that life-numbing trade off.

Q: Why should people want to improve the way they're living their life?

A. Rebecca: Because it's our responsibility. Because we are a country and modern society of people who depend on pills and have aches and pains and depression and obesity. I've learned that the most successful people in the world had somebody to hold them strictly accountable and then had discipline, something and someone really driving them. They didn't do it just because. It was usually somebody holding them accountable, challenging them and somebody enforcing a discipline on them that brought them to be where they are successful.

So I believe if we are not lucky enough to have that, we should do that for ourselves, we should be that for ourselves and then just imagine if we were all our own Rockefellers or Carnegies. I mean just imagine what the world could be if we all took it upon ourselves to discipline ourselves (even for a few short years) and get that level of success in our minds. Just imagine if there were more people in the world who were as motivated as those successful people were? I believe it is our responsibility to do these things and then help others do these things, and I will elaborate on that more later on in the book.

Q: Why should people learn authentic ways to cope and release stress do you think?

A. Rebecca: I feel like you're going to lose out more and more if you continually look to external sources for coping mechanisms. One day something is going to happen to you where you're not going to know how to cope with it and it's going to be so detrimental that you're going to have a personal tragedy, anxiety attack, heart attack or some other dis-ease. You know, why not prevent that?

Let's shift the focus from 'why not' but 'why should we?' If we focused on improving our coping skills and our natural abilities to handle things and make choices we can do so much more in so much less time that we will blow our minds with what we can achieve and our success. And that goes right back to the successful living and health and wellness all being combined.

So the more we focus on looking inward and our own skills for coping, we empower ourselves and so then again it goes into empowering our business, empowering our relationships, empowering our children, empowering the future, changing the world, being a good member of society, etc.

Q: How do you feel about prohibition?

A. Rebecca: I touched on that earlier and happy to reiterate. I don't agree with it because I believe that some people need those temptations, that path to get to their ultimate destination of right action. If they don't do it in this lifetime then it wasn't meant to be, but I don't believe taking away alcohol is going to make everybody happy, because what happened in prohibition was everybody went crazy, broke laws and that's not the way to do it. It's not the solution and it's not how I believe, even though I do believe that nobody should really use alcohol. I would love to see a society who chooses not to drink for coping or drink for celebrating and the alcohol just fizzes away from our humanity on its own as we evolve.

Q: How do you feel about AA?

A. Rebecca: I do not know a lot about AA. But what I know about it is that it is a strict faith-based and a 12 step program that sets pretty restrictive rules. One of my alcohol-free interviewees touches on how he felt his experience with NA (narcotics anonymous) was so restrictive, it just did not serve him. He was ready to change, and change he did, stayed completely clean. But he still hung out with people who were not and he still had success. I believe we need a system that honors all faiths and teaches better tools on how to mingle in society where everyone is on a different piece of their path and we can all coexist together without judgment. Once that program is established, I will be its biggest supporter. But there is a stigma around AA that I feel prevents people from going often. They don't want to be labeled "a drunk" or have their work or families judge them for it. So I think there are a lot of people out there who need help and just continue on without it. THAT is one reason why I created my movement called Clean & Present Movement. www.cleanandpresent.com

Q: How can people reward themselves in healthy ways vs. unhealthy ways?

A. Rebecca: The way that I've done it is the only way that I can pass along and it might not work for everybody, it might not work for a 300 pound 75 year old man who might have different interests, but what I love to do is reward myself through sympathetic nervous benefits like massage, Reiki, reflexology, hot tubs, gentle Yoga classes, relaxing in a bath with candles, slow walks in nature with no goal in mind, dancing alone and so on.

Another way to reward yourself is through like acupuncture, acupressure, reflexology, private yoga or ballet classes... Anything that can enhance your knowledge and connection to your body and it's sensations, anything that can relax your mind: getting your hair done, taking an art or music class, getting a facial, giving yourself a foot massage, taking an extra nap or laying by the ocean for an extra hour or making time and plans to lay by the ocean or a lake or river if you don't live near the ocean.

All these very simple things: taking a walk that is not intended for exercise but to go very slowly and look at the ground and the earth around you or the trees and not intended for getting somewhere. There's so many different things I could list and I will continue to list in the book on how to reward yourself.

Then each time you do something that's relaxing and working on improving the functions of your sympathetic nervous system you get more and more and more (it's a snowball effect), you get more relaxation, you feel better each time you get a massage, your digestion works better and you prevent depression. You feel that natural high that you want to achieve through alcohol and external forces, but now it becomes a reality in your every single day and multiple times a day. That's the trick, that is the solution, that's the goal.

Q: What is your opinion on the economy? People over extending themselves, spending...in relation to alcohol consumption?

A. Rebecca: I would say the economy that we've found ourselves in today, is the result of people who are buying things to make themselves feel better, though… I am the first to admit that I love nice things, for example, I feel like you should save up and buy designer purses and expensive hand bags because it's a better investment to purchase something, made by an artisan, one time, that's never going wear out versus buying cheap purses 30 times, that keep breaking on you.

I believe in luxury, feeling strong, nice and clean in clothes and I believe in quality things but I believe that there is a fine line between that, wise spending and over extending and I believe we've gotten ourselves into the whole thing that we've heard of, 'Keeping up with the Jones' thing because people are in that numbed state of alcohol-life-brain so that they are trying to find things to buy that excite them and that make them feel all those happy and relaxing feelings that we've numbed ourselves with alcohol from over the years to feel and we just don't feel naturally anymore.

So this vicious cycle is happening where we're over extended, we have credit card or school loan debt and we feel bad about it and the daily grind of work, trying to pay it off, keep up with the house payments, tired mind, stressed life, so we drink, and so we get worse and worse and worse and it's a snowball effect, that goes faster, in the wrong direction. That, I can go into in more detail later in the book but that's my basic answer for now.

Q: How do people feel when they have fun alcohol free?

A. Rebecca: So again it's that natural high that actually does exist, that is the goal. People, when they repeatedly breathe deeply, if they're hiking or doing a yoga class get a sense of euphoria that is better than any alcohol buzz and I know because I've felt it. I know because I've talked to people who feel it and it's not crazy, it's science and when you get a good amount of healthy oxygen in your lungs and fire your muscles nicely, you start to feel the serotonin expand in your brain, which is the feel good chemical. And you get more and more of it in a healthy lifestyle and that is good and fun. When you go to a large body of water... people like the ocean and often like being near water because large bodies of water release ions that trigger serotonin levels which is again, the feel good chemical in your brain. All of these things are free, clean and not involving drinking... which by the way is quite expensive when you price good liquor, wine or beer over a life time or even a year. Think of what you could save per year if you never bought alcohol?

You can't have those things happening when you're drinking, those things are subdued, those chemicals aren't released as much because when you relax yourself through alcohol you're also relaxing the functioning of your brain and your heart and every organ of your body flows along. Plus the body is just trying to regulate and process that alcohol and cannot do much else. Your liver doesn't work as well, with an alcohol life style, obviously, so the functioning of the body is struggling to make up for that and it's working hard to maintain itself, long before there's chronic disorder or disease in the liver or elsewhere.

So the body, just to get through the day, is just trying to survive, is just trying to withdrawal from the alcohol from last night or last week, just trying to stay hydrated. It's trying to detox from last night's binge, if it was a particularly "good" night out, it's just trying to balance itself and it doesn't ever get the chance to feel the fun that we can feel, like you would feel on a rollercoaster (if you like rollercoasters) or like you would feel at an exciting birthday party when you're eight years old. You know, you can feel those things as an adult -if you're sober.

Q: What memories are the best to have, or create?

A. Rebecca: So the best memories that anyone could have are an experience like, and I like to use the example of Disney World. When I go there with my daughter she tells people, when they ask her about her experience there, "What did you like about Disney World, did you have fun? Tell me about it?" She doesn't tell people about the glowing $10 Tinkerbell we bought for the fireworks show, she doesn't tell people about the ridiculously overpriced balloon I bought her, she doesn't tell people about the food that we ate - the soft pretzel that was shaped like Mickey Mouse, she tells people about how she felt when she got to drive her own car in a racetrack game.

She tells people about how she was scared in one of the rides that would turn the lights off and have one of the characters creep up on you. She would tell people about how it felt to meet the princesses and Goofy. She doesn't talk about what we ate, she doesn't talk about what we drank, she doesn't talk about anything that we bought; she talks about the way she felt and the experience.

So those memories that we have and that fun that we feel is all experiential. To me, a memory is created through being fully present, excited and feeling something in your heart and in your brain, and in your emotions and food doesn't do that for us and drink doesn't do that for us and buying stuff does not do that for us. Doing stuff, being active moving through something and being fully aware of it is what your memory remembers and creates love and happiness around. So if you spent every holiday, every birthday party, every vacation and every celebration numbing yourself through alcohol and closing your brain off, you're not going to have any happiness left in your body or in your life.

You're not going to have anything joyful, you're not going to have a memory of vacation; you're 'gonna have a memory of feeling hung-over. And your best memories are sober and through action of doing something and feeling it and experiencing and that is what life is and that's what it should be. So you're happier when you're more present and you're active.

Q: I love that Disney example! What is authentic happiness and why do you compare it to the feeling people get after winning a game or contest?

A. Rebecca: I like to tell people, "Okay, think for me what it feels like when you're the big winner of a contest or you're the winner of a game?" Just think about that for a second, how does that feel? That is authentic happiness. Happiness is when you have succeeded or you've gotten something unexpected or somebody recognized you and again, none of it has to do with buying anything, or things in general, it sometimes is just recognition alone. Sometimes just having your name called out in class or something, at a meeting at work or in a group of friends is enough for you to feel happy and so recognition, giving and receiving causes authentic happiness.

So the turnaround is, is that you should work really hard at doing that for other people because if you know how good it feels, and you know that that's what people appreciate and people like it and it causes happiness in their lives, you should want to help create it. And so automatically it's that snowball of attraction -thing coming back. If you feel like that never happens to you maybe that's cause you're never doing that for other people; maybe you need to think about how many times you've told somebody, "I appreciated that thing that you did." "I respect that thing that you did." How many times do you look up to something somebody did but you didn't ever tell them you felt so? I mean it happens more than you realize and so finding authentic happiness is also giving it because you would never have that authentic happiness if somebody didn't give it to you as well. So we must always feel and do both in order to recognize it and receive it, in my opinion.

It's sort of a circular thing, it has to happen - and again, it really can't happen drunk.

Q: Why should people focus more on getting a good night's sleep?

A. Rebecca: Okay so sleep is one of the things that keeps you lean, healthy and don't we all want to be a lean, mean, machine? Sleep, water and stress release are the top three things that prevent belly fat and belly fat is just about the number one thing that people try to lose when they start a work-out program or start working with a fitness professional. Not only that, so belly fat develops around our vital organs, visceral fat is around the most important parts of your body and so it's also the most dangerous fat to have on your body anywhere. And that fat, it starts to go away when we sleep a lot or regularly get the proper amount of sleep, your body stops storing that fat, to "protect itself" or store those energy reserves for later, since your body knows it won't have the adequate rest to do so, which just tells you how important sleep is. And I'm not talking about drunk sleep. We are not truly resting then. I am talking about SOBER, restorative, sleep.

When you drink alcohol your body is never fully resting because it's processing all of the acidic toxic stuff in alcohol, all those sugars it becomes and your body's working hard to process that so it's not sleeping fully, it's working hard to rid itself of that and to cope and to get back to its sober state. So people who drink every night have not had a good night's sleep in how many years? It's pretty scary and so look at how much they're probably not accomplishing and not doing. Even if they generally feel fine because they're used to that life, just think about what else they could be doing, accomplishing and could be feeling that is really so great that they're missing out on.

Also it keeps your brain working better, you get better test scores, you can do better at work, more promotions, you're more intensive, more intuitive... the list goes on and on and on. It is this recurring theme in the book; that snowball effect.

Additionally, the subject of sleep brings us to my biggest weight loss tip: I never eat after about 6pm at night. It might sound early. But if you eat high quality nutrients, good fats and tons of vegetables all day long, you really are not super-hungry after dinner. And I say, ALWAYS make dinner grain-free and early. If you have eaten foods void of nutrition all day, then of course you will still be unsatisfied and hungry all night long. I promise though, if you ate well that day, fueling your body properly to get through the day, then you are not hungry after dinner. And make dinner early. Then if you stop eating, let your body process it's dinner and food long before bed, it is not going to be working on digesting all night long when it should be resting, and your sleep is exponentially better for it. Each night I allow this in my life, I wake up and the scale is lower, jeans are loser, clothes more comfortable. It is my best tip for healthy, balanced living through weight.

CHAPTER 7
TOOLS, BREATHWORK AND MEDITATION

Q: How do you teach someone to breathe with control?

A. Rebecca: I teach people to use breath work as a tool to shift how their body feels as well as their mind. But teaching people to harness control of their breath can sometimes cause anxiety at first, but it can also prevent anxiety - which is how powerful the breath really is (going back to how powerful breath work is).

So what I do is I teach people to close their eyes and work on breath mainly through meditation and yoga.

Q: Why meditation?

A. Rebecca: I really believe that meditation is the one of the only ways, a magic key to a happy life and you can't really have a good meditation without having a clean and present body that's toxicity free... you can meditate with alcohol being a part of your life, but it's not very good. So it goes hand and hand with the clean and present movement and having happiness and loving your business, balanced mind, etc.

I feel like meditation is really the answer to so many questions that it's especially important nowadays because we're so over-inundated with digital phones, TVs, computer screens, billboards, advertisements, newspapers, 24hour news, news that has a talking head and scrolling in bits underneath and the stock reports on top, it's just like all too much! And so I think it's really important to go to a place that's dead silent and quiet and inward and that is when we almost effortlessly take hold of our purpose, our wisdom, everything. Things that feel so brilliant just come up out of nowhere when we just sit in silence as often as we possibly can.

I mean meditation is imperative, especially in this day and age. I couple it right along with each and every workout, at the beginning or end.

Q: How do you teach beginning meditation, or to beginners?

A. Rebecca: Well most of the time people say, "Where do you start if you've never meditated before?" I hear this really so, so often. So I guide people to a list of books, recommended texts which I list in the back of this book. But books by Ram Dass are great and I guide people to my website where I have free uploaded meditations for beginners (guided meditations), as well as ones for purchase, that can be really serious programs for beginners, for specific goals and achieving big things in your life. Found at www.taohappiness.com

It's a different brainwave than for example hypnosis - but, like hypnosis, you can meditate for achieving very specific goals in mind. And so for beginners I take baby steps and I really just consider meditation a sister or brother to prayer. I think prayer is basically meditation; meditation is prayer. I believe they are one and the same and so basically just starting with an active prayer practice or praying practice is often the very first step and then we build from there.

Q: What do you do with people who have anxiety with the breath work or they're feeling anxiety about breath work?

A. Rebecca: Yeah so it can be really scary and I am totally aware of that, and I've actually felt it before. When you try to control your breath in yoga in different techniques and different ways sometimes you get a panicky feeling because to control your breath means that you might not be breathing exactly when your involuntary breath would want to so it can cause a state of panic.

Like if you're holding your breath for too long, that can cause people to panic, just like when you are about to hyperventilate. But constantly knowing that you're the one in control of everything in your body and your space is such an important lesson to learn, that getting through that panic is easier than you think once you've gotten through it. And then you really are control of everything better in your life! It is awesome how that works.

It's almost like childbirth, once you've pushed through it, you realize 'Oh I can do that'. It seems impossible before it happens or while you're right about to go through with it or while you're in labor about to push, whatever it might be, but then once you do it you realize, 'I can do it, I did that!' - referring to natural childbirth.

It's the same with breath work, you know that there's nobody holding their hands over your mouth making you not breathe for that brief moment that you're taught to hold. So it is not exactly the same panic in that sense. For example there's a breath technique where you breathe in for four counts, then breathe out for eight and that eight counts is very long and it can make people feel panicky.

But I just suggest pushing through it and going forward with that sometimes scary and struggling feeling because again, the breath is sort of the doorway to heaven, it can bring you to a state of euphoria and peace and control in your life like you've never known if you just continually and patiently forge forward.

Rebecca Sweeney

Q: What should people do if they don't have time to meditate?

A. Rebecca: They should make time. It's the same as exercise. It's imperative and it's sort of like the balance to our overly visual life like I was talking about before. It should be the basis and foundation of your life, it should be as essential as eating or fitness in my opinion, just like a daily routine like brushing your teeth.

You can start to meditate at five minutes a day, so everybody can find five minutes. You can steal away to the bathroom while you're at work, you can find that five minutes. If you have five to ten minutes to crack a beer or smoke a cigarette, you have time to meditate. In fact, meditating is quite like smoking, a series of repetitive breaths where you get away, do something just for you and almost take like, an adult time-out.

Q: How do you retrain your brain and why do you mention this in your teaching?

A. Rebecca: Retraining the brain is complicated because our brains, I have been taught by scientists, actual people in the science industry, that our brains don't like change, they fight it. So when you're trying to change a habit that's why it's so desperately hard sometimes, or an addiction, because our brain does not like change, it's very hard to accomplish a rewiring or a re-firing of neurons that are used to going in the same pattern over and over and over again. But you have to remember that just like they got into that habit, they can get out.

So it's hard to change your brain and it's hard to retrain it but you can. Just like you got into a habit, it's just the same, you *can* get out. So getting into a habit usually is not a quick thing, it usually is a very repetitive thing that we do over and over and over again trying to achieve a certain result, then it becomes a habit - even if it's a negative habit and even when we don't realize that it is forming, we just do the same thing, only in reverse: -always moving toward the positive, for the GOOD, clean, healthy results.

Same with positive habits: So doing things over and over and over again, even if you think that it's not helping, it is actually rewiring your brain. You just have to remember that it will sometimes be difficult, possibly take a little while, but you ARE going in the right direction, so long as you never give up.

Q: Why do you recommend journaling?

A. Rebecca: Journaling is a tool that can really work through some serious stuff like when you can't figure something out or you're confused. The answer comes sometimes, just as in the quiet of meditation, sort of out of nowhere. Like asking yourself, why do I want this cookie when I know I'm not hungry and I know it's not good for me? I physically know in my frontal lobe, in my consciousness, that this cookie has no nutritional value but I want it anyway.

I offer just a suggestion to people who I coach to keep a journal in their kitchen for the weight loss issue, or maybe even an alcohol issue, whatever your 'cookie' is: your cake, your doughnuts, your alcohol. We'd normally say keep a journal there instead, walk over to it like you would walk over to a bottle of wine or a cookie jar and write; just brain drain, just drain your brain, don't write with punctuation, don't write with correct grammar, just write what comes up and say, "I know that eating this cookie would feel this or that," or "I know that drinking this wine would make me feel this or that and I want to

71

feel this because, and later it would make me feel...." And so on. Then see what you find!

I suggest right now, stop reading the book, and go and write, writing is releasing, list a bunch of words that you feel when you drink alcohol, the day after you drink alcohol, why you don't make fitness or money a healthy priority, how you hide from your emotions with alcohol or food, we all do it. Just drain your brain and list it. We do not focus on release enough! What are you having a hard time giving up that you know is not good for you, you know is not serving your best life? Your highest self? What have you not said to someone? What have you not made time for? What do you wish you could take back and are going to forgive yourself for? What are your goals? And what can you add to your life that will make it better and healthier? This should be a regular, scheduled practice as well.

So often when you write it out and look at it on paper, it's almost like you're taking it out of your brain and throwing it out, bringing it all into a neutral place. You don't even have to go through the ritualistic process of ripping it up and tearing it up or burning it and throwing it away. Just the writing starts the process of processing things you don't often think you need to address, but might be totally holding you back.

Just getting it all into a different form changes the energy from floating around in your head, swimming in confusion, onto a piece of paper and it takes you through these steps of starting to recognize what you're doing and why. In a way it organizes the floating, swirling, scrambled, monkey mind. It's really powerful and especially powerful to write knowing that you're not ever 'gonna read it again or maybe nobody else is and that it doesn't have to be perfect, it's just a drain and it clears your mind. It doesn't mean you have to cope, it's a coping mechanism itself and it's a tool to teach you about things you don't understand about yourself.

I was shocked when I once talked to a man who worked for NCIS. He dealt with the most horrific things. As did a family member of mine who was a paramedic and rescue diver. They both had to study and/or remove children, bodies and people who had perished in a scary and horrific way. I heard their stories. I asked the NCIS fellow, "did they teach you coping skills on how to deal with these images, memories and feelings?" He just said, "nope." I was so confused. For all the months and years of training these brave men and women go through, never once are they taught coping skills or tools. For people like those heroes and for people like office workers who slave to keep a large company afloat, people all around us, we all desperately need coping skills, or else alcohol is going to be our answer, whether we realize it or not.

Q: What are repressed memories and how do you deal with them?

A. Rebecca: Well repressed memories I just think it's important to bring up. -That sometimes we do things and we don't know why and sometimes we have memories that we've repressed and somebody once guided me to dig up what they believed I had repressed.

In my research, and this could change in the future (what I think and what I've learned) but for today, what I believe, is that repressed memories are repressed for a reason and nine times out of ten they usually need to stay there for some reason. And with that, there is a wisdom in our bodies that is greater than we know, because we don't know exactly how the Universe was created, so it is undeniable that there is a wisdom in the Universe that is greater than our awareness. I am a faithful believer in God and I just do not question some things. So don't try to dig it up if you don't know the exact details of why you do some things that you do, I would say.

You don't have to know, all you have to know is that you're in control of your today and your right now - and, in my opinion, you don't have to go back and relive a lot of it or drudge through every single bit of your past. Sometimes you *do* need to remember things like maybe go back and do an exercise about what upset you when you were six years old, that's fine and really healing to do, often. But if there's a repressed memory that you think could be causing you to act and have a behavior that you want to change, I just say to focus on where you 'wanna go. You don't have to dive into the past always in my opinion.

Q: Why only focus on good? Isn't that hiding from what is?

A. Rebecca: It's the opposition thing that I was speaking about when quoting Robert Kyosaki. Working in opposites is really awesome and life has evil, there is evil that exists in the world: there is negative, there is violence, there is bad - that's inevitable, it happens but dwelling on it is not gonna do anything other than expand it, and it expands the issue and expands the anger in your heart, just like the snowball effect I've been talking about as a theme recurring through this book. Usually evil is born from a lack of love somewhere. So what is the best way to deal with that? Focus on MORE love.

So not pretending like it doesn't exist, you don't want to do that, acknowledge then move along, but focusing on the opposite is just so powerful. So if there's negative - it's okay - it's there to teach us something and it's also there to remind us to be positive. You cannot see light without a shadow and you cannot see a shadow without light, so it all has its place and there's good and bad, and yin and yang, and dark and light, and hard and soft to everything, they cannot exist without one another. But I believe going in the direction of good and going in the direction of love is the only way, and it's not denying anything negative, it's just a direction like a compass in your life. Going in the way of bad, evil or tough, that leaves us exasperated and fed up at some point, eventually. Going on in the direction you believe to be genuine and good, does nothing but provide us an endless fountain of expanding energy and again, love.

I recommend NOT protesting for what's wrong in the world, but rather focusing on a similar subject or organization that is making something right, in the same realm. Protesting just breeds more anger in my opinion and we need none of that!

I recommend focusing all your energy on the political people who do not complain about others but focus mainly on the goals at hand and what they can control. All of these things combined with meditation, journaling, caring for yourself will virtually create a healthy body, mind and society, substance free, all on its own! Can you imagine if we all practiced this?

Q: Can people be healthy and also drink alcohol?

A. Rebecca: My answer is going to be in a question, because I have people, when I tell them my personal choice of drinking - that I don't anymore, they immediately tell me how much they do or they do not drink, themselves. "Well I drink alcohol but only like one glass every now and again" or "Well I'll go months without having a drink" or "I only have one drink a week or maybe once every few days and when I drink I really only have one or two." And it's like my question is, Well why do you even need that one? If you drink so seldom, then why at all? I mean really, why? To me it's just like saying I only have one cigarette every now and then. It is not needed.

To me, that's what I hear. It's something that's unhealthy for you and it doesn't really do anything for you so why do it at all? It puts a hurting on your liver, you know smoking is bad for your lungs so why even include it in your life? My question is just to get people thinking; it's not to say I believe everybody in the world should quit drinking.

I just believe, yes, you should consider yourself at your healthiest when you're alcohol free completely but I do know healthy people who drink and I do not judge them and that would be my answer to that.

CHAPTER 8
THE IMPORTANCE OF FITNESS

Q: Why do we need to exercise?

A: Sounds like a silly question, I know, but the people need to be reminded! We need to exercise for endorphins and for proper brain functioning and that's the main reason in my mind - to prevent depression. I think that's the most important reason among the many reasons, it releases things in our body that make us happier. –Bottom line. I think that we can say that happiness is a cliché. Oprah has said happiness is a cliché, that it's overrated, that joy should be more the goal.

I think happiness is: every human being exists on this planet to get to a place of happiness, whether it's the way that we think it should be or the way your neighbor thinks it should be - it's all different. But everybody wants to feel good, everybody wants to feel happy and comfortable in their life and body and skin and so exercise delivers that.

I believe that we didn't need to focus on fitness 6,000 years ago because fitness was what we had to do to stay alive. There weren't modern conveniences that we have now so it's even more important to focus on action and the body and I think it's cool to be in the modern world because we know now: -we know more about sports science and we know more about the way the body reacts to different actions and different reasons, so that's great.
I mean, we can control and do more and benefit our body more than ever before because of the knowledge that we have now and it's always getting better.

Fitness is, I would say, the second most important thing. It goes back and forth between fitness and meditation to me because your brain works better when

77

you exercise but I feel like your brain also works better when you meditate, so it's like the Gemini twins: you can't have one without the other. I believe they're so important that it's just vital to thinking, to your blood flowing, to your body functioning in every single possible way.

Q: Why should people do yoga along with exercise and why can't they just do one or the other?

A. Rebecca: People who only do yoga still have injuries or weaknesses and I believe that doing the same thing, whether it's a yoga practice that's really balanced, moving in every direction, utilizing every muscle, or baseball every single day - it's the same thing over and over and over and over again. Then it goes back to the that yin yang principle. I highly recommend Paul Grilley, he is one of the masters of Yin Yoga and creator of a phenomenal DVD Yin Yoga program that I believe everyone should do to be in a perfectly balanced body. Yin yoga focuses on therapeutically stressing the joints, not the muscles. This program also comes with a talk he gives about, "Why yoga?" He actually addresses from a medical stand point, *why* we should do yoga and how it physiologically effects all of the human body. His program can be found on www.pranamaya.com. He also offers a fantastic meditation tutorial DVD.

You need to exercise not only your joints but your muscles, so you need to exercise your muscles just like going to the gym and ripping your muscles with weights… it's important (a healthy stress on the muscles). Getting stronger is important, it supports your back, it supports your posture, it supports your brain; like I was just saying, but also your bones. In Yin yoga it works your bones, joints, connective tissue and it prevents arthritis more than just a typical yoga practice.

I recommend P90X, I'm such a fan of it because Tony Horton (the creator of P90X, P90X2, 10 Minute Trainer), he knows that you can't be a super buff body builder dude with zero flexibility before something's going to happen to your body eventually. You have to balance the body with flexibility as well as strength and so well rounded cross-training programs should be in everybody's mind, for life, just like sleep, eat and brushing teeth, doing all different kinds of exercise: (a) so you don't get bored with anything and you always stay active and healthy for life and (b) so you confuse the muscles and don't over exhaust your body in one particular way, repetitively.

Even in an Ashtanga or Bikram Yoga practice, which is very round and balanced and moves your body in a million different ways and is fantastic mental and physical conditioning, is still the same thing, every single day it's the same series over and over and I just think that you can have too much of one thing and it's good to mix it up. Our bodies really thrive when we do that.

Q: How are digestion and sleep affected by working out and in yoga?

A. Rebecca: Strengthening   the   belly   makes   your digestion work more efficiently. Abdominal work in exercise and yoga and the crunching type motion that you do with pulling your knee up to your chest in an asana or movement in yoga, twists in yoga, not only help your digestion –by tightening the abs up if you go to the bathroom too much and pushes it all through more efficiently if you get constipated or go too seldom- but also helps your spine and that's your nervous system, so every reaction and sensation of your body's signals to the brain work better, more effectively. So you use the food better that you put into your body, you use it, process it and get rid of it better when you do exercise and yoga - and, like I was just saying, how beneficial sleep is mainly for weight balance and maintenance.

Most people don't get enough sleep, that's proven. You sleep better when you're tired and you're tired after you do a really good work-out so you earn that sleep and that sleep comes easier, belly fat disappears, which also causes better digestion, etc. Especially people who are insomniacs or have trouble sleeping at night really need to do a good exercise and try that to start and see if that helps everything.

A lot of times when I have beginning yoga students in my classes they come back for a second class and they say "I cannot believe how well I slept that night after my first class." A beginning yoga student is like the most exciting thing ever and their sleep is phenomenal, well usually, when they start... and that's great, I love to hear that and I already talked about how important sleep is. You know, Doctors tell us, "you need to lose weight, exercise and sleep this amount and so on." But they never tell us WHY. Why do we need Yoga? Why do we need sleep? THIS is the why.

Q: Is there such a thing as too much sleep in terms of being healthy?

A. Rebecca: I think there is. I don't think an adult should sleep more than ten hours a day, I think that at that point you encourage sluggishness and you go past like a normal cycle of waking and resting that can turn your body reverse and you start to make life confusing and counterproductive.

Q: What if people hate to work-out?

A. Rebecca: This is a terribly common question! Usually it's the same in yoga as it is in exercise, usually the thing you hate the most is the thing that your body needs the most. The thing that makes us the most irritable and uncomfortable is the place within us that needs the most work and attention. So the people who hate it the most are usually the ones who desperately need it the most because your body doesn't always feel good when it needs to rid itself of something and working out works out cramps and toxins in the body, discomfort, disease and so if you hate it, I'd consider diving in full force and then eventually I promise you, if you stick with it and you stay positive you will look forward to it and it WILL become your majesty in life. The people who hate it the most are usually the ones who get the biggest, most miraculous benefit once they dive in fearlessly and stay with it.

I recommend trying many, many different fitness videos, classes, groups, private lessons, hiking, jogging, kayaking, climbing, canoeing, walking, running, sports, dance, anything until you find something you somewhat can stand and then continually move toward adding more and more accomplishments onto your list.

Q: You just spoke to me! What if people don't want to lose any weight?

A. Rebecca: So if people don't want to lose any weight, you don't do an intense program. I talk about this with clients every day and so this is going back to what my book was originally going to be about which was more like the fitness coaching that I've been doing for a while now. So I would just quickly say there are ways to stay active and physical for more of your mental state and chemical balances without getting too low in weight, that is so important, so you still have to know your body. But I'm not going to go into this too much because the direction of the book is now more guided towards **super** clean, sober living. However, people who are really low in weight usually need to build muscle and strength/bodily structural support so exercise in some way is for everyone, we just need to find your right path. Weakness is never healthy. Maintenance, if you are already lean, strong and balanced, is usually nice and enjoyable light exercise like every other day, so yay for those folks! Also nutrition is really important in those situations of low body weight, just as important as for those who have a bunch to lose. Protein and good fats, we all need that in our meal plans.

Q: Same thing to whether people have too much weight to lose?

A. Rebecca: If people feel they have too much weight to lose and cannot even contemplate beginning or getting it off, overwhelmed, then they just need to know that there is something for everyone and this goes hand in hand with a handicapped question, somewhat. Find your support, find your solution. It is out there. But just knowing that there is a way to move that doesn't involve hard jumping or impact on the joints; there's always a solution for everyone and I list on my web site, all the many solutions for people of different sizes, www.taohappiness.com.

Q: What if someone has a heart condition?

A. Rebecca: If someone has a heart condition of course talk to your doctor first and then obviously exercise is going to benefit the heart but you need to talk to your doctor first.

Q: What if people don't like to work-out inside and the weather is too poor?

A. Rebecca: A lot of times I get that excuse where they're like, "I like to run" or "I like to be outside only" and then it's winter in Ohio, so now what? There has to be a solution and so you have to get out there every single or every other day even if the only thing you like to do is ski and you work full-time and you can't ski every day, you have to find another solution: You have to get out in the rain, you have to get out in the snow if that's what you say that you do, you have to do it. We have to embrace a life where we don't find ourselves giving and living excuses.

Then you have to find that plan 'B'; it goes back to the plan 'A' that "Yep, I would love to work-out at this time or in this location but I couldn't today 'cause something stopped me out of my control, the weather can't always stop you, you have to find a plan 'B' in work-outs as well as plan 'B' time slots, as well as food choices, as well as everything. You cannot live by all the obstacles and excuses, you have to exist and thrive around them.

Q: What if people don't like to work-out alone and they don't have anyone to do it with?

A. Rebecca: Then that is where I would recommend again the shameless plug of the Beachbody community, they/we hold one another accountable. Community is so important in all of life. Also paying it forward was a big point I wanted to touch on. If there's something in your life you're lacking, somewhere you want more support, offer it to somebody else. Saying "I want fitness in my life…." Well, start a fit club! Community groups are huge. Mastermind groups are so empowering and actually get people better results quicker when they have a group of people working toward the same goal. So I say, create it if you don't have it.

Q: What if people can't afford a gym?

A. Rebecca: I will have a list of recommended online yoga classes, online fitness options and books that you can follow, recommended texts to self-teach. But also that is what I love about Beachbody, they support at-home fitness, it cuts down on the drive to and from, so many people are intimidated by gyms. But if you really want that exercise bike or treadmill and don't own one, go to the gym like the YMCA, it is usually affordable or offers guest passes. And then go hit it hard on an at-home workout plan. You have to make this a life style, a non-negotiable, no matter where you are, at home, traveling for work, working out in hotel rooms, it has to be in your mind as priority ONE each day you wake.

Q: What if you have a handicap or serious injury?

A. Rebecca: Obviously you want to let injuries heal safely in time, but handicaps should not ever stop you, neither should injuries - there are ways around it all and I will go into that more but also always the disclaimer: talk to a doctor first, find out what is approved and then most importantly DO IT. Wheel chair yoga classes are a wild success, for example. Find it, google it, do it.

Q: I think you already answered this but I'll just say it again: What if people are too tired or depressed to get up and do a work-out?

A. Rebecca: Yeah so thinking in opposites again is so important to remember and remind, however, I do want to recognize that I know how hard it can be when it feels impossible, I've been there. I have **been** there! So sometimes we don't even understand how we can even believe that we could ever even force ourselves to do it and that's where having other people, mastermind groups, accountability partners, coaches, fit-clubs are so imperative because having that discipline there for you when you don't have it for yourself, until you do, the importance of reaching out, giving it back and community, that's a huge aspect in my training. Self-talk is HUGE. We must talk our brains into believing in the impossible and the unimaginable. Then miracles actually do happen. Just google the name: Richard Neal.

A good example is in yoga. How do you think some of those super floaty, twisty poses are achieved? By practice, diligence and patience, of course. But there comes a time in all of our yogic practices when we have to talk to ourselves. Our mind becomes the thing that gets us into that free standing hand stand in the middle of the room. Yoga instructor Kino Macgregor (www.kinoyoga.com) taught me this. She mentioned in one of her awesome (free) YouTube tutorials to just tell yourself, "I bravely place my strong shoulders above my hands." -when doing an arm balance upside down. I mean, you have to talk to yourself. When you come to the thing you don't want to do, but know you should do, and just say, "I am going to do this and it is going to be incredible." Whatever you have to say, start talking to yourself. You have to go crazy to get sane, I always say.

Q: You are a big advocate for yoga for everyone, what if there's no yoga teachers or good studios in your area?

A. Rebecca: I do think absolutely everyone needs yoga. The new way I do yoga is very slow and mostly on my own. After years of "power yoga" and doing it all so super-fast, I do a really slow practice now. No more fast, it's what I recommend to most, make it fast, if you want to, after you have been doing it ten or twenty years, but until then it is beautiful and equally as good of a workout if you do it slow! Because the only way we can learn and improve our body is by deeply experiencing each pose and transition for long periods of time. If you go slow, sweat builds quite fast and it feels beautiful instead of forced, no exasperating. You really get to think in a long hold of a back bend/Urdhva Dhanurasana/wheel, "is the pose holding me or am I holding the pose?" These deep, life transforming thoughts translate to every lesson and discipline that exists in our life. It is that important for me to pass along.

But the "no teacher in my area" –thing, that was a big excuse of mine for a long time. Heck, I lived in Okinawa, Japan, in the middle of the Pacific for 3 years for Pete's sake, I had a pretty good excuse! I would say, "Well I only like to do yoga for my fitness, and there's no yoga studios here so I'm just 'gonna sit on the couch and get fat." That was me. So I wasn't motivated enough to do my own self-practice at the time for some reason, battling depression and sadness, being a pathetic military wife, no Whole Foods grocers on the island, I just gave up. And I was even a certified yoga instructor and knew what I was doing, so I'm not going to tell anybody else necessarily to do that but again -I'll list at the end, where I recommend some phenomenal on-line sources and home videos that we have easy access to nowadays that can help with that solution.

Q: What if your kids won't let you work-out?

A. Rebecca: Then I had that excuse as well! I relied heavily on that excuse as a young Mom. And now I've learned that if you don't work out during nap times, and you don't give the kids an option and you have patience with them and yourself, -like I used to feel scared to work out with them 'cause if I was lifting a weight and they climbed on my back I felt like they were going to hurt me or I was going to hurt myself or I was going to hurt them and I just got frustrated. But you have to just be prepared, be patient and continue because when they see you doing this and accept the practice as something that just is like we brush our teeth every day, we work out every day, then they let you - eventually they *will* let you. And it becomes magical for you and the kids both. My daughter just said to me the other day, "Mom, I want to be just like you when I get bigger." I mean what an amazing thing to hear! I never thought I would ever hear that coming from one of my daughters for some reason? It made me cry when I realized that. That was said after she pretended to do an Insanity workout like she has seen me do. So funny. What a far cry from me hiding my cigarettes and wine glass from her just a few short years ago. Amazing. You cannot even believe what they see and pick up on energetically. I would be proud today to see her try for the things I do. And that is my biggest gift as a Mom. Now I know it is actually imperative *to* work out in front of them, when I used to avoid it at all costs, because it frustrated me if they interrupted my program. But now I know they *need* it as much as I do! They need to see it, even if they aren't working out right with me, it is still planting a very beautiful seed in their brain and psyche.

A lot of times the big excuse I get is "My kids won't let me work-out," I used to really blast that excuse. But that is not an excuse because I've learned that because I made priority number one: my fitness and my love to myself, I've taught my kids to sit down right down next to me and they just say, "Mommy's working out right now."

I do it whether it's relaxing or not, whether I enjoy it not, whether it's the best work-out I could have gotten with or without them - I do it anyway. Over time they will let you do it because they understand it as an absolute just like the sun coming up and down. So it is a growing and learning process. And they soon let you do it, because it is boring to them, as that thing they are so used to.

CHAPTER 9
FABULOUS FOOD, DIET & NUTRITION

Q: What is the percentage and importance of nutrition in a healthy comfortable body, in your fitness routine and happy life?

A. Rebecca: So even though this percentage is here and exists as common knowledge, I still felt it more important to get moving first. However, as I got into it all I learned and do know for a fact today that nutrition is between and 70% and 80% of keeping a healthy, balanced and lean body. So it seems to be by that statistic more important than exercise but -sometimes you hear people say it's 50/50... nutrition and exercise go together 50/50. Well it's true too because you can't have one without the other, you can't lose weight and have a balanced body by just watching what you eat and you can't lose weight and have a balanced body just by exercising alone, at least not to your ultimate goal of perfect health or the best we can get. The two create a whole, they both get you to 100%. And you desperately need good food to have a good workout experience.

So nutrition, however, going backwards into what I'm saying turns out to be 70% of it, it's a little bit more effective than anything else in your weight loss journey, and what you put into your body is a tiny little bit more important than what exercise you've accomplished or the calories you've burned. So yeah, food, intake, that's a majority of the total, a big deal I think.

Q: What does nutrition support in your body?

A. Rebecca: Just as an example, I'll just throw one example out now and then I'll broaden it out more throughout the book, but just the mere fact of water representing our intake, or what water we take in, prevents soreness, lubricates and promotes suppleness of the muscles. Just drinking enough water helps you sleep better, helps your brain work better, improves your digestion, helps your heart work better, just water alone. Pretty amazing. So imagine our potential if we got the right amount of water and high quality nutrition every single day? Sad thing, most people don't ever get that.

So that shows right there how much it matters what we put inside of us, which goes back to alcohol which goes back to toxins in general and what effect it all has on our body and mind.

I started to get really serious about thinking about alcohol consumption from a nutritional standpoint when I did a cleanse system called the Ultimate Reset from Beachbody (www.myultimatereset.com/ZenMamma). It is a 21 day cleanse that is meant to nutritionally, physically and totally reset your body from a lifetime of absorbing toxins and pollutants. Also I saw people all around me in the wellness and fitness industry cleaning up their food, grass fed beef, all organic veggies, never eating peanuts or corn or any grains, going vegan and certainly no inflammatory foods. And then as soon as it was time to "celebrate" or "relax after a hard week," without a second thought, they just drown themselves in any old wine, fine or not, or grain based liquor or alcohol or beer. Do they ever take the time to question whether those grapes were organic? What pesticides might any of those production companies used in their wheat, barley, potato or grape growing process? There are not *that* many fine, organic wines. But the same people who desperately cared about not ever eating a piece of bread will without a second thought go and have a cocktail on a regular basis (ehem, this was once me too). Alcohol is very damaging to us nutritionally. It is loaded with empty calories and it is extremely harmful in inflammatory properties and brings a large acidic and sugar reaction to the intestinal system. But no one talks about this. Would you drink four glasses of grape juice one after the other? No. You wouldn't. Then you probably should re-think your wine intake. And I can already hear the "but's." They won't eat cake, but they will drink wine like it's their job. I did this, actually! And then I had to stop. And write this book! (laugh) I just want people to think about it all. A lot of people just don't for some reason. There is a grey area with health, wellness, alcoholism and this culture. I think we need to look at it. This book is here, in existence to examine and bring up the grey area to everyone's attention.

Q.: What does nutrition really do for you or support in your work-outs?

A. Rebecca: You can get more accomplished in a work-out with what you have eaten before. So to repeat, you can get a better work out and get better results from the work you put in with what you eat beforehand because it's giving you more efficient fuel for your workout and then the amazing thing is also that you have about an hour after a workout to consume a certain amount of proteins to help repair and recover your muscles at an accelerated pace. Food is so amazing with how what you take in, it can drastically affect the way you give to or accomplish your work outs as well as recover from your work outs.

Q: What is "clean eating?"

A: I think Tosca Reno the author of the *Eat-Clean Diet* and all the clean eating cook books coined the term and clean eating is what I use as a part of my description of the movement that I created that I really want people to jump on, have meetings and groups about, spread the love, share the recipes, motivation and so on. It's sort of like total clean living; recycling, clean and sober, and clean eating - all go together in my mind, it is a lifestyle and it's just eating, being and living whole. I really respect the Straight Edge movement that started a while back, for being the same way, or similar in some aspects. In the Clean & Present Movement we're not eating anything that has preservatives in it or chemicals in it, hormones or antibiotics for mass produced meat or any food that was boxed or bottled up by somebody else in a factory and broken down and added stuff in it to keep it fresh in that box that makes it to your pantry. It is cleaning up everything. Being more in control of your life, starting with your choices.

Clean eating is whole food eating, making things for yourself, so if you want ice-cream you make it yourself, if you want french-fries you make them yourself and you know every single ingredient that went into it so you're not eating anything toxic. You're keeping your diet very clean - very, very important. If you have not seen the film Food Inc. yet, I really believe every single person needs to see that film.

That's why I don't understand why there are nutritionists and people who go out and picket and fight the company who doesn't deny GMOs and who will only eat organic and only eat vegan but then they'll go and buy whatever bottle of alcohol. They don't often know anything about what's gone into it, they don't know anything about the fermentation process or how it's going affect their body tomorrow or next week, but they won't eat a grape if it's not organic. It just completely confuses me and I'm here, again, to bring attention to that in all of us.

Q: What do you know about preservatives?

A Rebecca: I know very little about preservatives, I'm not a nutritionist and I'm not a doctor but I have a gut feeling, in my own little world of studies that I have done for myself, that preservatives are a major cause of disease in our body. Just what my gut says.

Q: What do you know about hormones and antibiotics in our food?

A. Rebecca: It would be the same thing. The same answer as above, exactly.

Q: What if people can't afford to eat healthy?

A. Rebecca: This is a super-hot topic for me. This is one thing that I've disagreed with some leaders who I follow as far as finance and budget. And second, I believe if we give it enough effort, we can find affordable and healthy food sources and solutions. I feel like I could sit down with anybody and tell them one or two things to exclude including cable TV, including a higher car payment, including an iPhone… whatever it might be that I would sacrifice before I would sacrifice eating healthy foods. However, I have a long list on my website's blog (in the Insight tab on www.taohappiness.com) of ways to eat healthy in affordable ways. Tips and tricks on how to save money and still eat organic and clean. I think it's more important than cable TV. I think it is more important than smart phones. But do people want to hear that? It makes my coaching job kinda' hard! Cuz, no. Most people want to hear none of this! But check out www.Bountifulbaskets.org, food co-ops and places similar who are supporting farmers markets and saving people thousands of dollars and making it really easy for us to eat better for cheaper.

Q.: What has changed in your life regarding healthy food?

A Rebecca: I saw my weight loss accelerate and everything snowballed when I took control of my intake and started educating myself: the people I hung around, the success in my business, the happiness in my life, the happiness in my children, the health of my children, the behavior of my children, all drastically improved when I focused more on nutrition. The behavior of my children in school: big, big difference when you feed them well, that's a huge thing in our life.

Q.: Yeah?

Q.: What diets have you tried?

A. Rebecca: Every single diet in the world. (loud laugh)

Q: But can you list some?

A: Yeah, well I don't really recommend counting calories, I don't really recommend counting carbs, I don't recommend counting points of any kind, but that's just for me, it works for some people. And if those work for you and you are perfectly happy with your body, you probably don't need this chapter! What I'm talking about is what works for me in this book and counting is something that I'm eventually going to get irritated with, give up, fail out and I don't want people to fail, I just want people to eat clean, whole foods.

I started out with starving myself occasionally in high school, I was never anorexic but I would go a few days where I'd barely eat and love how my jeans fit, but then your body goes into starvation mode and packs on the pounds to protect itself, so that was a vicious cycle that I think most teenagers go through. I'd love to prevent that by educating them how that starvation mode happens and then back fires on us.

Then in college I was like a carb loader, I just got addicted to carbs which led me to the Atkins diet. And that diet makes weight fly off my body, but in the Atkins diet if you even begin to look at carbs again, even healthy carbs, you gain it all back and then some, so you can't really have cheat meals in that plan. I'm a big fan of cheat meals, I think everybody needs them to stay happy and balanced. I eat pizza about once a week because I flippin' love it.

So the Atkins diet lead me to the South Beach diet and on and on and on and on... I did the "Abs Diet," the weight lifting diet, the slow carb diet, I've tried every single diet and none of them worked until I just recently grew interested in the Paleo diet. I'm sort of on a Paleo kick but I don't see it as the end all be all and I combine it with healthy low fat dairy and I can also direct people to lots of good diet choices for beginners in nutrition on my YouTube page and on my blog from the website here: www.youtube.com/taohappiness
www.taohappiness.com/news

Q: How do you not overeat when you're really, really hungry?

A: Yeah, so that's almost impossible. Humans by nature have insatiable cravings for fat, salt and sweet just to fill up, so just remembering rule of thumb: (1) drinking tons of water keeps you feeling full - a lot people know that as well... but a good thing to try and get used to remembering, is grabbing a glass of water when you think you want a snack, try to re-train your brain to immediately think water, and drink an entire glass of water, and then think about how you feel? If you still want that snack then eat it because you are authentically hungry. But if you don't feel hungry, nine times out of ten after you've had that water, your body just wanted something and water could have been the trick and you don't feel hungry anymore. Then you walk away and go about your life without having that unhealthy snack or whatever you craved.

And remembering that (2) cravings and overeating are our body trying to get something that it doesn't have so it's almost impossible to fight - so don't fight it but try your best to eat things of substance and I can list at the end of this chapter here what foods of substance are. When we drink alcohol and when we eat processed foods, filled with preservatives, our body wants more and more and more and more 'cause it's trying to fix all the toxins that we're bringing into it, so it's trying to heal, it's trying to satiate it, it's trying to feel satisfied and we never do so it's a vicious cycle so we just keep eating more and more and more and more junk food -that's how people, that is how almost all of us get fat.

But the good news is that you can eat as many vegetables as you want pretty much; you can find a way to make a vegetable soup, veggie stir fry or make a smoothie or make something vegetable-based where you can eat as much of it as you want. And like Dr. Atkins says (that I really like), you can never sit around on a couch and pop too much steak in your mouth, like you physically can't do that like you can with potato chips, or you cannot eat bacon all day long but you could eat potato chips or pretzels all day. So you just think about food in the whole form and think about it in the vegetable and the healthy form and you can eat as much as you want.

Q: How does eating right prevent depression? How is the stomach involved?

A: So there's been theories about how the stomach is where our happiness is born and the focus on clean eating in the recent years has been a very, very big testament to the fact that if we eat right we're happier and if we exclude heavily processed foods and crops that are over-cropped liked grains... grains used to be wholesome and healthy for us but are over-cropped these days, they're over-processed, they're overgrown so there's a soil depletion so there's no nutritional value in a lot of grains and even vegetables these days. So I'm not a big fan of carbs for that reason because they're void of nutritional value and so I believe that certain forms of gluten and certain forms of grain can cause depression. I think avoiding most processed foods can prevent it and actually make us feel happier and you can look into studies on why they have gluten free diets for autism and it'll show you the same thing. How those kids and those people thrive on gluten free and grain free, clean eating diets, well then why don't we all just eat that way then? - is my question. Obviously what we put in our stomach affects our brain. Again, just something I think we should all just *look* at.

Q.: How often should people eat junk food or cheat meals or desserts?

A. Rebecca: A good tip from a man, a creator of one of the fitness programs I've done, Insanity, his name is
Shaun T, said you should "write a list and on the left side write all of the foods that you love that are healthy foods and on the left side write all of the foods that you love that are junk foods and then make 85% of your diet the healthy foods on the left and leave the rest for some of the junk foods. Because you're not going get fat eating a bag of peanut M&Ms you're not 'gonna lose a bunch of weight eating all the foods on the junk food side." So you need a balance, it's just the yin and yang we've been talking about; you just don't need a lot of junk food, you can't let

yourself indulge all the time but that 85% is a really good tip from him that I follow because it keeps us sane and it keeps us from binging or going crazy with too much restriction.

Another good tip is from the Okinawan diet plan. When I read a book about their diet and later got the awesome chance to live on the island for three years, I saw that the only time they eat sweets or junk food is on very, very special occasions Like only for your own birthday or weddings, that is all. Otherwise, it simply is not a part of their life style. Maybe one reason why they have the most centenarians (people who live to be 100 or more) out of any other culture on earth. They also eat a lot of sea vegetation and sea food, which is *not* depleted of nutrients, like our soil is. The run off of soil into the sea keeps the ocean vegetation and fish filled with trace minerals and nutrients we need. Eat your sea veggies.

Q.: What is the difference between the way we eat now versus the way our grandparents ate?

A. Rebecca: When our grandparents ate a bowl of spinach, to compare to us, it now takes about five bowls of spinach for us to equal the same amount of nutrients that they got because of the earth's current soil depletion I mentioned. So the way that we have to eat now is very different from the way our grandparents ate (and I can go into more detail on that but I just touched on it).

Q: What are super foods?

A. Rebecca: Super foods are the solution to that soil depletion in our diets, they are rare foods that we're finding and collecting in certain corners of the earth like the foods found in the drink Shakeology, created by Darin Olien, www.darinolien.com. Shakeology turned my health and natural energy and workouts completely around. I used to make super food shakes on my own that cost tons of money to buy all the ingredients separately. I would buy spirulina, sea weed juice, chia seeds, flax seeds, aloe juice, green tea matcha powder, protein powder, kale, other veggies in bulk, etc. and fruits to make my own juices and smoothies. Shakeology replaced and included all of that for me for a fraction of the price. You can find super foods in health food stores now in their raw form, in energy bars, in powders. But if you want to make it easy for yourself: get on Shakeology like now and watch your life blossom. You don't need to worry so much about having 9 servings of vegetables each day when you do shakeology and you feel like a re-birth, a whole new, amazing life. Super foods are essential to us all in this day and age. To learn more about shakeology and how I can help you with this vital nutrition source, check out www.myshakeology.com/ZenMamma.

Foods of Substance List:
(What to go to when you feel like you cannot control cravings. These are foods packed with nutrients and/or to prevent cravings)

-Kale, steam it for 5 minutes, throw some sesame or olive oil on it and some Himalayan Pink Salt, maybe some curry powder, put it on the side of every dish!
-Avocados
-Hard boiled eggs
-Tuna fish salad with celery and mustard
-Granny Smith Apples
-Raw Almonds or Cashews, handful
-Mangos, fresh or dried
-Plums
-Melons
-Berries, grapes
-Kiwi
-Hummus (try and make your own, super easy)

-Cucumbers
-Salmon, get some in a can if you want to keep cost down
-Snap peas
….just to name a few….

-List of recommended text fall at the end of the book.

CHAPTER 10
LIFE AFTER ALCOHOL, NOW WHAT?

Q.: What are people's biggest fears when they quit drinking?

A. Rebecca: People's biggest fear is, "I'm not going to have fun anymore." And, "What do I do when people ask me, why I'm not drinking or why I quit alcohol? I don't want to be judged or labeled." Basically I touched on this in the beginning but I have to reiterate: that it's never as big of a deal as you think it's going to be, socially.

When people ask you if you want a drink and you say, "No thank you." They often don't even care why. You think they're gonna care 'cause you care but they don't care. They just say, "Okay." And they go to the next person and ask them if they want a drink.

Everybody knows somebody who doesn't drink and they don't really think too much about that person's choice. So it's never as big of a deal as you think it's going to be. And it's absolutely not true and I'm just here to tell you that you're still going to have fun, in fact you're going to have more of an authentic fun, like I talked about. -Like you feel when you win something. Or like you felt when you were eight years old at a birthday party -the kind of fun that comes back to you and it's going to be your life and it's more fun than getting wasted. I just promise it. Especially if you make "fun" one of your core values and expect it and create it for others, it absolutely materializes and it is way better and way more fun than falling into the front door entry way of a fancy bar from your too-high heels, with too much to drink, at the age of 32, straight onto your face. (yea, I did that)

Rebecca Sweeney

Q: What do people think when someone doesn't accept a drink that has been offered?

A. Rebecca: They don't think anything. Again, we think they're going to judge us and think, "Oh, they must be an alcoholic." But just think about what I thought of the people who didn't drink who I knew back when I drank? I thought the opposite. I thought, "wow, those people must be so amazingly healthy, I want to be like them." Or people don't think anything and I've been told that by multiple people. So clear your mind of that worry, if you are making this choice for yourself. And if you *do* happen to come across people who give you a hard time if all of a sudden you are choosing not to drink, or skip going to bars with them anymore, chances are some people will lash out. Some people, out of their own toxicity or jealousy, might give you trouble. And I am going to get really real and tell you right now, no matter how good you think that old friend is: YOU DO NOT, IN ANY WAY, NEED THOSE PEOPLE IN YOUR LIFE. They do NOT serve you and your highest good or support your reason for being on this earth. So let them go, you do NOT need to be in their pity party-misery loves company-world. You're welcome.

Q: What does it feel like to be sober?

A. Rebecca: It feels relaxing, clear, healthy and clean and vibrant and amazing and closer to your source or closer to God, depending on what you believe.

Q: What can you do once sober that you could not do before?

A. Rebecca: Sleep better. Focus better. Patience. I think I did touch on all of that already. Am I a perfect picture of a Mother? Not by any means. But I am *way* better as a sober Mom. Oh! You can drive. Not make mistakes, not say things that you regret, things that you can never take back. You know, living with no regret is a beautiful thing. You can influence people, be a better leader, all of those things.

Q: How do you have fun with people who drink?

A. Rebecca: You laugh with them. You still are present with them, you don't judge them, you still enjoy the same things, dancing, singing, playing, joking. You still, you know, make your own personal choices and let them make theirs. If you feel uncomfortable with the level of alcohol people are drinking around you or the demeanor, then you remove yourself. But you just go about life being present and enjoying it with full awareness and without judgment.

Q: What is the O.A.R. technique or OAR, that you have mentioned helped you so much?

A. Rebecca: Yep. It's an acronym. So it's called the OAR technique and I was taught it by two friends who are life coaches. And this is the technique of: Observe, Accept and Release. It's a technique and a tool that you can use to get through any situation.

   If you're having a hard time saying no, when you want to make the choice to not drink or work through a hard time. You sit back and you observe how you're feeling and why. It is just called conscious living. Ask yourself, "why am I wanting this drink right now?" And then sit with the answer or until the answer comes, BEFORE drinking or before pouring that drink. Almost talking to and answering yourself in third person and then you will go through acceptance and accept that you feel this way, whatever it is —you accept it no matter what. It's just like being present with your pain. If you feel something painful, like I said in the beginning and you just sit with it, just allow, sometimes, before you know it, it just releases. The desire floats away once you have given it a title or given it a name or organized your reasons why. Often just this simple process is enough to get you through the toughest things that happen in our brain, I have found.

So often, the release phase of this problem-solving technique is usually the easiest, it happens on its own. It's just a technique you can use if you're struggling with quitting drinking or making healthy choices. I walk people through this is a guided, faith-based format on my web site, www.taohappiness.com.

Q: I really like that.

A. Rebecca: Cool. Yes, thanks, me too. This is just a way that barely breaks scratching the surface but can really help some people, I think. We all need tools.

Q: Why should people who barely drink or do not consider themselves alcoholic, give up alcohol?

A: So I just want to make a challenge to every reader and every person who I come in contact with, that if you don't have a problem with alcohol, just why not try giving it up then? Why not try living this empowered life? And seeing what it has to offer and seeing how you can help people in this way.

Just by, like the Ghandi quote, BE the change, starting with yourself and changing the world, why not try it? I challenge each and every reader to just play with that in their minds and see what your fears are, what comes up about why you wouldn't want to do it.

"You must be the change you want to see in the world."
Mahatma Gandhi.

Q: How do people let loose or let go without having alcohol?

A. Rebecca: It's silly to a lot of people, including myself, but dance is a sacred gift and a sacred movement that we can bring to our body to unlock things that are very locked up that we didn't even realize. It is the ultimate way to relieve a tight spine or back muscles or weak abdomen.

It's good for your core and spine which is good for your digestion and nervous system, once again, happy life tools. Yoga, all these things free the body and different closed up parts of the body, pieces of you that have been hiding away since you were little and much more free with play and confidence before you lost it at some point. Breath work and meditation obviously I recommend too, but mainly dance and celebration; alcohol free.

Taking classes like adult ballet, belly dancing, Hawaiian or Mexican style, take an African dance class or - I'm not sure even what you'd call Indian style dancing and maybe you could tell me...

Q: Like Bollywood dancing or something?

A. Rebecca: Yeah, like Bollywood dancing and just to move your body in a way that feels freeing. This is a looseness that beats the pants off of getting loose with alcohol because it not only makes you feel the euphoria that you would feel from drinking but it makes you healthier physically. The dancing has an aftereffect and this one is a benefit; it makes you stronger, healthier and it opens up closed parts of your body. Have you ever seen a professional dancer who doesn't look uber-fit and happy?

If you do not feel comfortable taking a class, dance alone! Dance in the shower, move your hips around in a warm bath tub. This rotates the spine and wakens natural energy springs that we all have waiting inside of us! We need this! When you are home along, just break out the candle stick microphone and dance. Make it a priority.

Also getting crazy. Like, joining groups of hang gliders or mountain jumpers, mountain biking, marathons, bungee jumpers or mountain climbers or, you know, healthy thrills. Exploring things that scare you in healthy ways. –These are much more exciting and wild, exhilarating and freeing than drinking or partying.

Q: Can I ask you to look at a perspective of mine, to that if you don't mind…?

A. Rebecca: Sure!

Q: I'm really self-conscious about my body and my weight and I would often, and still do sometimes, will drink alcohol so I *could* dance because I was embarrassed to dance otherwise because I didn't like how I looked, didn't like how I felt when I moved. I didn't like what people would see if I moved. And I loved to dance so I would drink alcohol so I could dance. So that was what I wanted to know, what you would say to that?

A. Rebecca: One question that I ask people who want to determine whether they have a substance abuse problem or not - not to pinpoint you but, is: do you use alcohol to be better at something? For instance, better at golf or better at singing or braver at dancing or singing in front of a crowd?

It's one reason to sort of look at what you are drinking for and that's a great thing just to self-explore and journal about. But the answer to that question would be, I would do stuff like, at home, that's why I'm such a big fan of home fitness and home workouts and doing it all alone because I dance by myself.

I even get a little embarrassed if my husband comes in the room and he's my husband. I do like, videos like ballet and salsa-type videos that are dance exercise and it's like, I don't want anybody to see that. But the more you do it and the better you look, the more you want to share it with people, like in fit clubs and stuff. Because I'm like, look at how comfortable you can get, look at what you can do just by doing this thing by yourself, then in public, sober, eventually.

I just believe it's sacred to move in that way. It does wonders for my spine; my back problems. So I would suggest starting alone then you automatically start losing weight and you feel better and you can do it in front of people, at parties or clubs or wherever without so much alcohol.

Yeah. It's a process it is a practice, it is slow, but it's like the wisdom from the book, *The Slight Edge*, the tiny little pieces of that all add up to one big thing that will eventually - if you definitely use it as a goal and stick with it, you can free yourself and do and feel and look the way you want.

Q: Cool. And, yeah, no worries about pinpointing me, I'm very well aware that I use alcohol for these things and I'm ok with admitting that! (collective laugh)

Q: Okay, what if people slip up or fail, how do you decide to have a life with one hundred percent no slips?

A. Rebecca: No, yeah, its personal to everyone -is just what I wanted to leave people with is that; it doesn't have to be my way or an exact science. What's, my way has worked for me, it's what I share and because of the fact that I did want to start a movement and a way for people to look at life differently today. Makes me say, I don't ever want to drink again because that would be bad of me, as the creator of this big thing. It was motivational for me to help people and also a way of holding myself accountable. I am all about doing everything you want to do publicly.

At the same time, I don't know if I'm going to say I'm never going to have another drink for the rest of my life. I don't say that and I would say to people, the reason I chose to quit drinking, the way that I did it was publicly. I used to always, you know, I would say to myself, for years, "I'm not going to have any more drinks, after this I'm done." And I would just make it a quiet decision within my own mind.

And then my husband would bring me a bottle of wine home after work with him on a weekend and I would drink it, of course. Because I hadn't told anyone. I hadn't shared with anyone. It is a taboo subject, not an easy thing to bring up or to consider with people. I hadn't held myself accountable or responsible in any way shape or form. And so I kept failing.

I just decided to start a movement for the fact that, I don't want it to be *me*, the movement about Becca, Becca created it. The movement should be about the people and people coming together, supporting one another's journey and creating their own little groups of community support of fitness, wellness, clean living, touching base, forum, support and gathering community in a clean and positive way   and   holding   each   other   accountable. (www.cleanandpresent.com)

When you do claim something that you want to do, publicly, you really do achieve it more often. Because you know that you said it and so does the world. Maybe the world doesn't care as much as you do but you still said it and you want your credibility to be good. You want people to take you seriously.

So blogging about things, becoming a part of the movement, talking to people about it, creating healthy groups. It's a great way to maintain goals but more importantly, I just don't think people should hate on themselves if they do have a slip up or if they decide, with a good mindset and good planning, this night is gonna be one night I'm going to drink for this reason____. And as long as they know it's good, with pure intentions and as long as they know it's not because they're trying to release stress or use it for coping then I think it's fine. It is just what I no longer choose to do.

Q: How do I find friends who don't drink?

A. Rebecca: Pray. When I decided to change my life and wanted to focus on fitness, I got down on my knees and prayed and meditated that I just wanted to be surrounded by a group of people who were positive and focused only on health and wellness.

I realized I didn't know any of those people and that all of the people in my life are actually the opposite of that. That upset me and I wanted a different thing. So I made the decision for myself to do that and then I thought, "How the heck is that ever gonna happen? I don't know where to begin 'cause the only people that I look at who are super fit and healthy, I don't have anything in common with it at this point. I can't go hang out with them doing what they do 'cause I can't do those things." So I felt very confused and lost and like I was like falling to my knees in desperate prayer. Because I just wanted health, super fitness, strength, happiness and friends to share that with.

Less than a week after that I made that prayer, I met my Beachbody coach at a swimming lesson that our kids shared. A place where you would meet someone who you might not have anything in common with but meet them, and chat with them, just the same. I believe it was God coming into my life and answering my prayer. My coach and her fitness world became the company that I work with now. I thought it was, again, a Divine intervention or my prayer answered because she had a community of people just like I then created with hers and just like I want more people to create. Small groups, it doesn't have to be "you're changing the world," just small, tiny groups, one by one, by one, by one. Then they'll change the world, not form one person, not from you but from many people, all of us, collectively. I asked for a community. I got that prayer answered tenfold. Life has never been better. So just ask for it, for exactly what you want, in detail. It always comes.

Having those small close-knit groups, having friends who you say, "I wanna lose 10 pounds." "You wanna lose 10 pounds, I wanna lose 40." "You wanna lose 40... let's do this together." Be the motivator so if you don't have those people in your life, you be that person to your friends. And the ones who come with you are meant to be and the ones who don't, you don't worry about. They're on their journey and it's just as good.

So be the leader, start that club, if you don't already have somebody who's asked you to join them.

Q: What should people busy themselves with?

A. Rebecca: Healthy things. The busier you are the less you snack, the less you want, the fewer the cravings you feel. If you busy yourself with self-help books, fitness, obsess over healthy recipes, and healthy things and projects that inspire you and books that challenge you- and workshops that are healthy and advance your career, you don't have time anymore to do the unhealthy stuff, or to eat unhealthy or to get into things that aren't good for you.

Q: How do people focus on being happy without driving themselves crazy?

A. Rebecca: There's a really good quote that I heard at some point, along the lines of, "in the pursuit of happiness sometimes we just need to stop and be happy." I was not a happy person for a very long time. In fact, I didn't have, what I would consider to be a happy childhood. I was pretty much unhappy my whole life. I am not sure if it was chemical or depression, lack of exercise or what?

But knowing that, I created a website and a business called The Art Of Happiness. Because I realized I needed to do the opposite, just like I've been talking about this whole time. I realized, I need to do what I don't have. I need to create something that I don't have, something that I want and I need to focus on it. It needs to be the name of my business because of what I am not.

And eventually it, my happiness, just happened on its own, I think because of that. So if you're not happy just call yourself a happiness warrior. If you don't feel like your friends are happy, positive people to be around then **you** be that happy positive person for them to be around. And just by the law of nature, happy things will start happening to you, good things will start coming to you. Good people will start being attracted to that good, that you're showing the reflection of in you - happens.

I know that because I'm a parent. Children are like little mirrors they hold up in front of your face every day because they do exactly what you do. So you cannot deny that the law of attraction exists. What you do compounds. It's just the way nature grows. We all have got to just know this by now, as total fact. Do what you want. Bam-you get more of it.

Q: How do people pay it forward or help others?

A. Rebecca: I already covered this but so essential to reiterate, it is fit groups, neighborhood volunteering and community groups. I don't think perfect health and balance can happen in your mind, life and body if you don't include selfless giving, or giving that you don't get paid for. In yogic philosophy they call it Seva. Also I think your results of your own goals and happiness speed up exponentially when you help others along as you are also working to better yourself. It is one reason why I think the Beachbody coaching business is so rapidly successful among members and as an LLC in general.

Q: I think you may have covered this but I'll just say it: What is the importance of showing people the importance of appreciation and how often should people take time to show appreciation?

A. Rebecca: Yeah, I did that earlier but it is one of the sources of authentic happiness. Gratitude should be a huge priority on our to-do list. Just list all the things you are authentically grateful for at least once a week. We all just need to feel grateful. We all just want to feel acknowledged by our parents, by our friends, by our loved ones, by our spouse. And so if we're not feeling that way, we should do more of it, obviously, to others and then it will always come to us more. Which feels really good. Who have you thanked today? Haha.

Q: How do people worship God more in their life, if they're not an atheist?

A. Rebecca: So I would say if you're not an atheist, I believe that spirit is a big part of this; spirituality, prayer, like I've already talked about. The word God has come up several times throughout the whole thing. But I do not recommend strict spiritual rules like in some recovery programs. Just seek your peace with spirit and worship and make it a priority. I don't care what brings you peace, or how you do it. But just definitely do it. Do yourself some good. It automatically will be bringing more good to the world. And I try to practice my worship, prayers and meditations, seven days a week, not with just one visit to church on Sundays.

If you're an atheist, I just suggest praying for yourself. -Life, honor yourself, obsess over yourself, glorify yourself, focus on yourself. If you don't have a God that you pray to, pray to yourself. Pray to the people who you love or have loved. Pray for peace in their life just as simple as a good intention going out of your brain.

I have been challenged on my meditation and prayer thought forms and teachings. I just want to address it briefly. Some religions teach meditation as a negative thing and it is most certainly not, because you're in control of what you allow in and out of your life and you're mind. I don't really believe in anyone else being able to control your mind. Things don't happen to you, you create it, in my opinion, so meditation and prayer can never be a bad thing, no matter what religion you are. Maybe that just can help a few people who are concerned.

Q: So why did you write this book?

A: I sat to write this book because of my own personal journey. Whenever something good happens to me I feel like I immediately have the response, that I have to share it with somebody, and as many people as I can. I always feel that way about beautiful things. That's why I'm in network marketing, because it comes naturally to me to want to share successes.

When I started doing yoga, I was so excited about it, I eventually, I felt like I just had to be a yoga instructor. And so it's the same for the book. I want to be able to tell people who are like me, I'm very normal; I have very much struggled with alcohol and food and toxic things in my life. I know that there's people out there that just need somebody who's down to earth who can say, "This is where you start." And that's what I wanted with this book.

Q: What concepts do you want to share with your audience?

A: The biggest concept is to think big. And by big, I mean, expect more for yourself than you can even conceive, your wildest dream, go beyond that. And in that way, sobriety is the key. So think big as far as -that's a big change for a lot of people. To think about never drinking again; that's huge.

And even if you don't decide to do it today or in two years from now, just tell me that you'll start thinking about it at least. That's the only seed that I want to plant.

Q: What do others say about you? Peers, clients, etcetera?

A: I have a list of testimonials from people who've told me that I really helped them with my guided meditations and my yoga instruction. I will share those and some more incredible interviews that really blow your mind, just awesome information to absorb and digest.

But what I'm most proud of is that people, this honestly is my most proud nugget, that people have come to me and told me that they were a beginner in yoga and in part through studying with me have become interested to become a yoga teacher as well and they've become yoga teachers. So that makes me happy, that makes me really, really happy. The ultimate spreading of peace and paying it forward right there. I want to go now and learn from those three or four people!

What I'm also most proud of is in my network marketing business as a team leader, when I helped somebody become financially free or independent or contribute to their household, if they're like a stay at home mom, and become the bread winner of their house, or helping someone who absolutely hates their job and wants something better for themselves or their kids and they get that dream in their hands through income in helping others get healthy, that is probably more rewarding than helping somebody lose 100 pounds.

Q: What do others say about the book?

A. Rebecca: I've had a lot of wonderful and exciting support from my network, and my friends in this project. I think people are proud of me that I'm pushing myself out there on a limb and doing scary things.

I have gotten just a very few individuals who are brave enough to say, you know, addictions are problems and people need to talk about this more- it's a taboo subject or it's hard to talk about and people do need to just do it.

I don't know if this is going to be a really wildly popular thing 'cause I don't think people want to hear a lot of it really. But I hope it lands in the right hands at the right times.

Q: Who is this book for?

A. Rebecca: I hate to say it because our workshop leader (Alicia Dunams) told us not to say this! -But this book *is* for everyone. I mean this book really is for everyone -but I'm going to, obviously, connect most with people who are around my age and have gone through what I've gone through, to some extent. So, stay at home moms, military wives, work from home and entrepreneurial women and people who have also struggled with weight, addictions and depression and who want to deal with it naturally. Also the thirty-something's, I am you, they are me!

Q: Who is this book dedicated to?

A. Rebecca: I will re-type this out and reiterate it from the beginning to the end. This book is dedicated to anybody who has had a struggle, a struggle that is so debilitating they don't know if they can get out of bed in the morning. They don't know if they can ever forgive themselves. They don't know if they can ever talk about their past. They are embarrassed of their weight. They are embarrassed of their choices, current and past. Has felt pathetic in their drinking habits. Who has struggled either with an excessive weight issue or struggled underweight with an eating disorder or just feel awful in their body. Anybody who has dis-ease in their body who's been so

strong but they're not sure there's a solution for them…
I'm here to say that there is.

Q: Why are you qualified to write this book?

A. Rebecca: Why am I qualified?

Q: Yeah, who are you and why are you qualified to write
this book? What are some credentials, awards etc.?

A. Rebecca: I can say that I am qualified for sure,
mainly because I have overcome my own addictions,
health concerns, and am sober and I've healed my life
naturally. And because of my own personal struggles,
weight issues, coming out of them on my own, naturally
and successfully, with my own victories, I also feel
completely comfortable helping others with theirs'. I feel
qualified working with people on an emotional and
physical level because of my over twelve years' experience
of yoga certified teaching and my nutrition experience in
the supplement and fitness industry for over a decade.

I have been in network or relational marketing for
over ten years. I feel that my self-motivation is reason
enough for writing this book and being qualified. But I am
also really qualified in helping others with home-based
business, because of my own business that I've developed
from the ground up.

Rebecca Sweeney

THE DIVINE INTERVIEWS
(Part 2)
& TESTIMONIALS

Interview #4

Testimonial #1

"I have done lots of guided meditations and Rebecca's are my favorite. She imbues them with a blend of grace and humility that really resonates with me."
–Hewitt Huntwork, Singer/Songwriter, from Laurel, Maryland

Q. Rebecca: I appreciate you giving me a testimonial for my meditation instruction, Hewitt. You have been a valuable part of my web site meditation development. So I wanted to expand on that testimonial a little bit in the book, if you would be so kind?

A. Hewitt: Sure!

Q. Rebecca: So how did you come upon my meditations and why did you stick with practicing them?

A. Hewitt: I saw your guided meditations advertised on a mutual friend's spiritual group facebook page and we connected there. I liked your unassuming style, the one where you held your baby when she would not settle, where you just showed up where you are with what you have! I am turned off by "guru speak." You spoke down to earth and it makes meditation better to work with. I learned once that "the truth exists in the language you already speak."

Q. Rebecca: Thank you! Yes, from yoga instruction to meditation, more importantly, I like to speak to with very plain language so anyone can feel it and understand. So thanks for the feedback.

So how do you feel about the book subject I am writing on?

A. Hewitt: Oddly enough, I am interested because it's funny, I was 39 years old before I ever had anything alcoholic to drink. Then, I went on a cruise when I was 39 and just decided to have a margarita! I used to have a rigid stance on not drinking. I was the only one who ever actually listened to the no-drinking health class stuff. Also, I knew the founder of M.A.D.D. (Mothers Against Drunk Driving), the Mother who had her son killed. It just made me not ever want to drink alcohol.

Q. Rebecca: Incredible! Oh my gosh, I had no clue you did not drink alcohol! I also cannot believe that you as well as my other testimonial are both musicians. All these parallels keep happening with this book! So do you drink now since the margarita?

A. Hewitt: I drink alcohol now like one time a month or so, randomly.

Q. Rebecca: Why did you start to meditate?

A. Hewitt: I was an angst-y, pre-artiste in high school, I was anxious, couldn't sleep and so I got a guided meditation tape from my Mom which I listened to and it actually just helped me sleep. But then I came back to meditation when I felt anxiety, I felt drained with life and work. What helped with this was affirmations and meditation practice. It keeps me from letting my own moods and emotions -from working against me.

Q. Rebecca: That is really great.

A. Hewitt: Yea, the most profound insight in why we

should meditate, for me, came from reading *Into Thin Air* by, Jon Krakauer. It is a book about climbing Mount Everest. And he says you know, mountain climbing drives out anything that takes your focus away from the task at hand, or else you won't survive. So he said that when he was at the top of Mount Everest everything else in his mind just dropped away. Because it is dangerous if you get distracted and are not totally focused on what you need to do to climb and stay alive and make it. It narrows your focus and I just compared this to the work toward meditation. The climbing and meditation, it both commands your attention and demands your attention. It demands your focus. And all other stresses, any other meaningless details in life, out of our control, just drops away.

It is like cross word puzzles or doodling also. Time flies when you get absorbed in a single pointed activity and it just calms your brain and prevents anxiety. That is why meditation has been so important to me, to balance my emotions and life through the tough and stressful times that are sometimes hard for me to handle. Meditation is so valuable to me for those reasons.

Q. Rebecca: That is one really fabulous way to explain the point of meditation to beginners or people who wonder why meditation is so good. I love that climbing analogy!

So do you have a comparison to talk about life without alcohol versus with alcohol?

A. Hewitt: You know one of my voice teachers was super strict. He made us fill out this detailed questionnaire and one of the questions was, "Do you drink alcohol and can you abstain from it?" His point was that it is a diuretic and keeps you from retaining water which not good for your vocal chords and singing. So I always remembered that too and live by it. I drink so rarely, really that I don't even consider myself a drinker. If I come across some friend's homemade mead I really will enjoy that. But not otherwise do I often drink. Occasionally at festivals. But it is a total non-issue to me and not a part of my life style.

Interview #5
(kept anonymous, initials M.B.)

Q. Rebecca: Thank you M.B. for doing this interview! Our mutual friend told me you should be interviewed for this book and I knew we had connected with my "giving up alcohol" blog post, but I had no idea you had actually given up alcohol until our friend told me! Congratulations. So when did you actually quit drinking?

A. M.B.:   Well, I tried to quit several times. But this time was successful on March 25th, so it has been about one month now. I had been deciding for a long time. I actually chose an on-call career where I could not drink at all. I always tried to be a moderate drinker.

Q. Rebecca: Why did you decide to quit?

A. M.B.:   Well, my father was an alcoholic. I kept hearing all the time in my head, "I am killing myself. I have a problem." Then one night I had a really scary thing happen. I was sleep walking. I had company staying at my house, which of course meant: drinking. In the middle of the night, I walked out and laid like face down, in the middle of the family room floor, totally passed out. I had absolutely no recollection of walking out there and doing that. It scared me when I woke up and figured out what had happened and I had absolutely no recollection of doing it.

And then I started to have panic attacks. I am not sure if you have ever had one? Your vision gets weird, it is a weird experience. It happened to me at lunch once, I decided then to not drink anymore. But that night, I had two beers. It was like my easing myself out of it because you know, I was addicted to it. But from then on out there was no more drinking.

I had night sweats for like, three nights after that. I wanted to drink again but I was actually afraid to.

Q. Rebecca: How did it feel a little while after you quit, to be sober?

A. M.B.:   I enjoyed sleep better as a sober person. I enjoy waking up. But I get sad, lots of crying. I really miss it! For me it is a coping mechanism. I am going through divorce, it makes me feel normal when I drink. It sounds weird, but being a Mom of three, it is the only thing I do for just myself.

Q. Rebecca: So interesting to put it that way, it makes total sense. And how do you feel today?

A. M.B.:   Right now I am a midwife student only. And I am honestly toying with drinking as a student before my job responsibility starts. I would never drink knowing I would be on call for someone else's birth. But I can drink, do it for myself now, while in school. Oddly, the instructor showed us a bottle of liquor in the classroom one time! I thought, "oh wow? They drink?" It made me think of just drinking while being a student. But I have not.

Q. Rebecca: Did they offer you a drink that day? And if so, what did you say?

A. M.B.:   They did, and I just said, "No thanks."

Q. Rebecca: So how do you cope now?

A. M.B.:   Actually, I have an anonymous blog about being a sober Mom that gets like over 300 hits a day! It is really amazing, it is very popular and it really is a great way to vent and release and feel supported and support others.

Q. Rebecca: I think that is totally wonderful. Do you mind if we share the name of that blog since you have written it anonymously?

A. M.B.:   Sure! It is titled *Super Mom* -like tongue in cheek kinda' thing, *Super Mom Gets Sober*, www.supermomgetssober.com

I also cope with rap music. (laugh) Artists like Macklemore, he is a sober rapper. His song called Neon Cathedral, it is a song about not drinking, it is amazing. I don't know if you have heard of the rapper Kendrick Lamar? He has a hit about not drinking and that music, music and rap about being clean really, really inspires me and is empowering. I get really into that.

There is a lot out there online for support as Moms if you look for it, you should check out www.cryingoutnow.com, it is a site about Moms who are dealing with recovery. It all helps.

Q. Rebecca: I love hearing your story. It is like none of the rest and that is why I think it is so important to include. Thank you so much for sharing everything and all of your wonderful story and information. So valuable!

Rebecca Sweeney

Interview #6

Testimonial #2:

"Becca is a natural teacher who knows how to give clear and down to earth explanations to any level of student without sounding preachy. She is obviously very passionate and knowleagable about yoga and pulls from a wide variety of styles and influences. Her classes are always varied and interesting with just the right amount of challenge. She was my first yoga teacher and inspired and influenced me so much that I eventually went on to become a yoga teacher myself." –Lauren Lapointe, musician/yoga instructor from, Savannah, GA www.laurenl.com

Q. Rebecca: Lauren, thank you so much for your testimonial and contributing to this book of mine about living a sober life! I know you are really busy.

A. Lauren: I don't mind at all, funny thing, not sure if you are aware of this but I don't drink alcohol.

Q. Rebecca: *What?* I had no idea! I cannot believe this. The other friend and client testimonial interview of mine was also a singer-songwriter and I never knew, as well as he was a non-drinker for most of his life. I am totally blown away! (big laugh) When did you decide to quit drinking alcohol?

A. Lauren: It was a gradual thing to quit consuming alcohol. You know I got into music late in life and I really consider my music following my bliss. Drinking is a big part of the music culture and I am also from Eastern Canada where there is a big cultural drinking trend as well. Also I currently live in Savannah, Georgia where drinking is a thick part of the culture here as well! But I really felt as though, in my music, alcohol kept me from being fully present, gives me an edgy feeling. And I feel that when we find our path, our dharma, we just don't need the tools that alcohol provides.

Q. Rebecca: That is totally crazy, because the movement I started because of this book and my new life direction, is called The Clear & Present Movement and it is for pretty much that exact reason that you just mentioned! The coincidences are just all over the place with this project. Incredible. So back to you. What do you do now when people offer you a drink, what do you say? I know it is all around you in your environments.

A. Lauren: Well often at a gig people will sometimes feel moved or touched, feel something from my music and they will come up after and buy me a shot or a drink. And I just learned that you cannot get all nervous and make a big deal out of it because then they sense that awkwardness. I just have no stress around it and say, "Oh thanks, I never drink when I play." So people don't ever see it as a big deal. I would just rather go in clearly and be fully present with my music.

Q. Rebecca: So how do you relax and stay centered and fully present with alcohol not being a part of your life?

A. Lauren: I do yoga, eating well, I stay alcohol free (which helps), meditation, breathing and breath work. I center myself before a show with this little ritual, I go back stage or into a bathroom or something and take three consecutive deep breaths before all shows I play.

Q. Rebecca: How do you deal with social or celebration experiences involving drinking?

A. Lauren: Most of my friends do not drink. My partner/husband does not drink, so that is nice. He just doesn't like it, it is as simple as that. Never has. But I do have a disclaimer: one time a year I will have a drink on my birthday, every year. We go out for margaritas as tradition. But then the next day I always feel horrifying! So I always wonder why I punish myself when it should be a celebration of myself? Really it feels like actual poison in my body.

Q. Rebecca: When did you become a yoga teacher and why?

A. Lauren: I got certified in 2009, so it is four years now I have been a teacher and I am adding to, upping my training hours now with Kripalu. You know when you find something you love you just want to share with people, after you have done it for a while.

I get a sense of giving with yoga, it is a nice balance for my music. They are both about being **on,** in a sense, and connecting (performing). And the more you get your own "stuff" out of the way, the more you connect with students and be your true self. I really love it.

Q. Rebecca: Thank you for sharing your awesome self with us. I cannot believe how well this fits into the book. I just planned on asking you about your yoga testimonial from a year ago. But this turned into an alcohol interview like my first three! I am so grateful for you.

Interview #7
Jamila Tazewell, Designer + Owner at 11:11 Enterprises,
www.eleveneleven.net
Q. Rebecca: When did you decide to quit drinking alcohol?

A. Jamila: You know there was not actually one moment that I decided to quit drinking forever. For me it was a very organic process of evolution. I used to drink very heavily and for many years. Like a lot of people I grew up very shy and insecure and found alcohol as a way to just let go and have fun. Sometimes way too much "fun". It was a big part of my identity actually. I really liked to get extreme and even kind of macho with liquor because everyone always thought I was so innocent! I loved pushing my limits and was basically a black out style drunk from my early teens till about the end of college. I had some really bad experiences my senior year that made me see that I really needed to change my relationship with alcohol. I wasn't thinking I needed to quit forever but I realized that I was really hurting myself and that needed to stop. I would say I became more moderate in my approach after that just from making that decision. Also I moved to New York City and realized that in a place like that I really needed to keep it together.

Fast forward a few years, I move to Los Angeles and I'm 26 years old, drinking here and there and smoking a fair amount of pot to relax. I start noticing that I am really not feeling healthy and I am having extreme anxiety. I start really getting into the classic California-type explorations. I start cleansing and juicing and doing yoga DVD's all just trying to feel better. I start seeing results. Then about a year into that process I am introduced to Kundalini yoga and at that point my whole health discovery process really took a quantum leap forward. I started doing a daily meditation practice on my own around that same time and it is at that point that I stopped drinking (and smoking pot) completely.

Q. Rebecca: And why did you decide to quit drinking alcohol?

A. Jamila: So I found that just by raising my energy frequency with the Kundalini practice, I started feeling so good that I had no desire to drink or do drugs. I literally felt (and still do) that my practice was getting me so high that alcohol and drugs would actually ruin my buzz! This is a pretty big deal for me to say because I was VERY interested in the buzz I was getting from the substances.. When I had the experience that I could actually create even better feelings naturally it was like a eureka moment! I can get high AND be helping my whole being be more healthy and strong? Sign me up.

Q. Rebecca: What has your life been like, felt like since omitting alcohol totally?

A. Jamila: Well I've continued to explore the ways that a Kundalini yoga practice can change me, and since that kind of yoga works really fast I've been going through a LOT of changes in the last 7 years. Not drinking and doing drugs has just been one part of the journey and to be honest I never think about what I "gave up" because what I have gained in terms of energy, awareness and enjoyment of life just trumps any experience alcohol, etc. EVER gave me... and I really used to love to drink so that's saying a lot!! I really feel like if I had a drink right now it would be the biggest buzz kill. There is no desire any more for it. I never thought that would be possible but it is true.

Q. Rebecca: How do you respond/handle it when someone, somewhere offers you a drink?

A. Jamila: You know I hardly ever have to decline a drink because I'm rarely offered one! I just politely decline like it's not a big deal... because for me it does not feel like a big deal.

Q. Rebecca: Second part to that last question, How do people react who drink, when they know you do not drink?

A. Jamila: I don't get much reaction to it because I think either most people I am around know I am a yoga teacher and so would assume maybe that I don't drink? My identity is not about being a party girl at all anymore so it's a total non-issue for me and anyone I seem to be in contact with.

Q. Rebecca: How do you celebrate? (at weddings, holidays, occasions, etc.)

A. Jamila: All the social anxiety I used to use alcohol to cover up is gone. I have no problem letting loose on the dance floor or whatever. I didn't even drink at my own wedding. Our guests had champagne and we toasted with Martinellis sparkling cider! haha! The joy I felt that night was so high and amazing that alcohol was the last thing I wanted to consume. Alcohol is a downer after all. I think my experience isn't anything too unusual either, anyone could make this shift if they want to. A big fear people who like drinking have is that if they become "dry" (such an inaccurate term!) that they won't have any more fun. In my experience the exact opposite has happened-- and if it can happen for me it can happen for anyone!

Q. Rebecca: Namaste Jamila, from the deepest part of my heart. Thank you so much for your time and sharing!

More Testimonials

"I have just completed my first week of P90x and Rebecca has been with me daily. Always giving me the right amount of encouragement and support when I needed it she seems to have a knack. I look forward now to working more than I've ever done in the past. Thank You So Much Rebecca!!"
–Steve Tredget, Toronto, Ontario

Rebecca Sweeney

"I completely lucked out when I met Becca! In just one class I realized all that I had been missing from own yoga practice. She filled the room with so much energy and peace at the same time that I wanted to become a yoga master for weeks afterwards. It always cracks me up because she is super passionate about her business and fitness in general, where as I am more laid back, and yet she works with me at my pace, never making me feel guilty or lazy, just answering my questions and showing me a stretch here or an exercise there. I feel very blessed to be able to call her a friend." -Christy Higby, Augusta, GA

"I was in an exercise slump when my sister introduced me to Rebecca. Since then, I have felt like I have a workout partner...many workout partners! I feel as if Rebecca is always close by...she always responds to each comment, question, or concern I have accountability, support, and I am loving exercise so much more now on her team than I ever have!" -Rebecca Gast Boehm, San Diego, CA

"Rebecca Sweeney is a dedicated coach with a heart centered approach to supporting her clients in their health goals. She caters to each person holistically and thoughtfully, considering all aspects of their physical, mental and emotional health. She is currently coaching me through my first Beachbody challenge and her knowledge and support have been invaluable. I look forward to more challenges with Rebecca and Beachbody in the future!" - Ali Iwaskow, Louisville, CO

"I had the pleasure of meeting Rebecca Sweeney at Gunner's Fitness Center in Okinawa, Japan at a morning yoga class I was teaching. I teach many varieties of fitness classes, so I would meet many people daily. However, I remember when she first walked through the door of class, hair pulled back in a tie-dyed headband, and rolled out her yoga mat for class. She was pregnant with her youngest daughter and glowing with smiles. This chance encounter was the beginning of a lovely friendship. I have had the privilege of watching her grow. (Yes, physically watching her tummy grow!) I have further had the privilege of watching her shrink. Oh, I don't mean just loss of her tummy after her daughter was born – I mean pounds and pounds of extra weight, as she sweated, sculpted, and nutritionally nourished her body to where it is today. Her knowledge of yoga, fitness, and nutrition knows no bounds, as she is always expanding and experimenting with new ideas.

My personal favorite thing about her style is the love that centers on every intention she puts into her actions. As yogis, it is a blissful state to love every moment and love your body to nourish and build – not hate into a stressful weight loss that is short lived and forced instead of embraced. We both have witnessed individuals wrapped in plastic sitting in the sauna trying to sweat the last couple or fifteen so pounds to make weight for the military! She literally decided NOW would be the best time and the best years of her life, and proceeded forward to make her dreams into reality. She started Beachbody to transform her own life, but she was unable to keep the secret of such a wonderful program. Thus, before she even knew it, she began transforming the lives of those around her and those that wanted the happiness she radiated. She is an amazing coach, spiritual leader, and an inspiration to everyone. She is continually online providing guidance to those is coaches, and always inspiring new ideas. I am grateful to have such an amazing presence in my life working for wellness and beauty in our society." -Erica Castor, MA Health Promotion Management , E-200, 500 – RYT, ACE Personal Trainer/Cooper Specialist and Beachbody Coach

Recommended Texts by Author

Business

-*The Next Millionaires* by, Paul Zane Pilzer

-*Rich Dad Poor Dad* by, Robert Kiyosaki

-*The Slight Edge* by, Jeff Olson

-*How to Make One Hell of a Profit and Still Get Into Heaven* by, Dr. John F. Demartini

-*First Steps to Wealth* by, Dani Johnson

Health, Wellness, Weight Management

-*Women Food and God* by, Geneen Roth

-*Master Your Metabolism* by, Jillian Michaels

-*The Eat-Clean Diet* by, Tosca Reno

-*Women's Bodies Women's Wisdom* by, Christiane Northrop

-*Bring It* by, Tony Horton

-*Journey of Awakening: A Meditator's* Guidebook by, Ram Dass

Recommended Fitness Programs from Home

-Free Beachbody coaching with Rebecca Sweeney: www.beachbodycoach.com/ZenMamma (just click JOIN and select the FREE option, multiple programs to choose from in fitness, cleanses, supplements and nutrition) www.myshakeology.com/ZenMamma www.myultimatereset.com/ZenMamma

-Reflexion Yoga, Online Yoga Classes in Your Home, on Your Schedule, At Your Pace: http://reflexionyoga.com/

-Wide range of a beginner Yoga DVD selection at: www.gaiam.com

ABOUT THE AUTHOR

Rebecca graduated from the Savannah College of Art and Design in Savannah, Georgia in 2001 with a Bachelor of Fine Arts degree in the Department of Illustration. Along with art, in college, she submerged herself on the crew and rowing team. This was the birth of her passion in fitness. She was selected to study with the college abroad in Provence, France, Florence and Venice, Italy in 1999. There she studied interior and exterior illustration.

Immediately after her college graduation, she became a certified Yoga teacher/instructor. Moving from the Yoga mat and professional Illustration world, she found peace in freelance artwork, creating custom art works for clients and constantly developing collections of multiple meaningful art series'. She celebrates her style changing and evolving constantly, which is going against the grain of the typical illustrator. The freedom in her work is inspired from her over twelve years of teaching classic Hatha Yoga worldwide at various Yoga studios.

Rebecca's biggest passion in life is to be a motivational speaker, combine art, creativity, wellness and fitness into helping people with their inspiration, health, balance and happiness in their own bodies, spaces and in their lives. She strives to bring the peace she sees through Yoga and meditation to her business. Rebecca aims to evoke continually positive reactions to all who view or own her art or to who become a part of her coaching team. She is the creator of TAO Happiness and The Clear & Present Movement:

www.taohappiness.com

www.clearandpresent.com.

Aside from running her at-home Beachbody wellness and coaching business, Rebecca celebrates peace, balance, equality, Motherhood, womanhood, nature, nutrition and diversity in every one of her artistic and business creations. Her passion above all, is to teach people how to love themselves once again, as she feels we all tend to lose the self-love we are each born with.

www.ingramcontent.com/pod-product-compliance
Lightning Source LLC
Chambersburg PA
CBHW051420280526
45785CB00003B/1101